Joint M

Date Due

OCT 09 2007			

BRODART, CO.   Cat. No. 23-233-003   Printed in U.S.A.

For Churchill Livingstone:

Editorial Director (Health Professions): Mary Law
Project Manager: Derek Robertson
Design Direction: Judith Wright

Joint Motion
Clinical measurement and evaluation

Roger Soames BSc, PhD
Senior Lecturer, School of Biomedical Sciences,
University of Leeds, UK

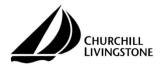

CHURCHILL
LIVINGSTONE

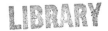
CHURCHILL LIVINGSTONE
An imprint of Elsevier Science Limited

© 2003, Elsevier Science Limited. All rights reserved.

The right of Roger Soames to be identified as author of this work has been asserted
by him in accordance with the Copyright, Designs and Patents Act 1988

First published 2003

ISBN 0 443 05808 3

British Library Cataloguing in Publication Data
A catalogue record for this book is available from the British Library

Library of Congress Cataloging in Publication Data
A catalog record for this book is available from the Library of Congress

ELSEVIER SCIENCE your source for books,
journals and multimedia
in the health sciences
www.elsevierhealth.com

The
publisher's
policy is to use
**paper manufactured
from sustainable forests**

Printed in China by RDC Group Limited

Contents

Preface

This book brings together the principles involved in measuring and evaluating joint motion and the underlying joint anatomy, to give an appreciation of the structures involved when determining joint movement. One of the problems associated with examining joints and their movements is that it is done through an intact skin; thus the importance of understanding the anatomy of the joint in question. It is not the intention of this book to be an authoritative text on all aspects of joint motion, but rather to provide a framework within which to work. The ranges of motion reported by others have been included, as well as the age-related changes. However, this information has been simplified to provide ranges of a motion that are required for specific tasks or activities, thereby enabling an immediate assessment of whether an individual is capable of performing the task or activity.

Section 1 gives a brief introduction to factors that may influence movement and the need to be aware of what is actually being measured. However, the majority of the book (Section 2) is concerned with the individual joints of the upper and lower limbs and vertebral column, as well as the temporomandibular joint. Each begins with an overview of the basic anatomy, followed by an account of the ranges of movement possible in each plane, together with the age-related changes where appropriate. This is followed by an account of the examination and measurement of the individual ranges of motion.

I hope that you find this book a helpful adjunct to an appreciation of movement and joint motion, whether as a student, clinician, practitioner or someone with an interest in how the body moves.

Roger Soames, 2003

Acknowledgements

This book has had a long gestation period, for which I am indebted to Derek Robertson and Mary Law of Churchill Livingstone for their patience and encouragement. I am also grateful to Tim Lee for taking the photographs used to illustrate the text, and to Helen Armstrong-Brown for being a very willing subject. Any errors or omissions within the text are mine.

Roger Soames, 2003

Section 1

1 Joint structure and function

INTRODUCTION

The bones of the body articulate at joints permitting the controlled movement of one bone with respect to another. The joints of the body can be grouped into well-defined classes depending on their structure, with the type and extent of the movement possible depending not only on structure but also function. The classes of joint are fibrous, cartilaginous and synovial, with fibrous being the least mobile and synovial the most. In both fibrous and cartilaginous joints the articular surfaces of the two bones are joined by connective tissue, while in synovial joints the articular surfaces are not directly connected.

The majority of the joints of the appendicular skeleton (i.e. the limbs) are synovial, the exception being the inferior tibiofibular joint where the bones are joined by a fibrous interosseous ligament: the axial skeleton displays all classes of joints.

SYNOVIAL JOINTS

In contrast to fibrous and cartilaginous joints, synovial joints are freely mobile, being linked by a fibrous capsule. The opposing surfaces are covered by articular cartilage (a specialised form of hyaline cartilage) or fibrocartilage of varying thickness with contact being between the cartilaginous surfaces only: movement is aided by the presence of synovial fluid. Some joints contain intra-articular structures, such as menisci, ligaments and tendons.

Articular cartilage

Articular cartilage has a distinct zonal organisation (Aspden and Hukins, 1979), with variations in cell type and arrangement, architecture and calcification at varying levels from its surface. It has a wear-resistant, low-frictional, lubricated surface, is slightly compressible and elastic, being ideal for movement over a similar surface, as well as being able to absorb large compressive and shear forces. In large joints in the young articular cartilage thickness may be 5–7 mm, being smooth and compressible, whereas with increasing age it is thinner, less cellular, firmer and more brittle with a less regular surface.

The articular cartilage is moulded to the underlying bone, with variations in thickness often accentuating the bony surface contours (Fig. 1.1).

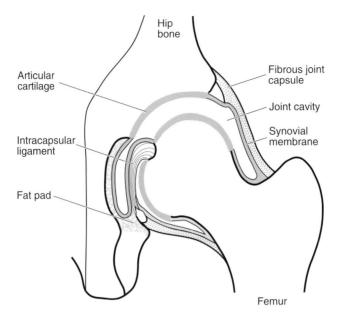

Hip bone

Articular cartilage

Intracapsular ligament

Fat pad

Fibrous joint capsule

Joint cavity

Synovial membrane

Femur

Fig 1.1 A synovial joint showing the articular covered joint surfaces, fibrous capsule and lining synovial membrane: this example has an intracapsular ligament.

Convex surfaces tend to be thickest centrally and thinner peripherally, while for concave surfaces the reverse is the case. It is both avascular and aneural, with its nutrition depending on a peripheral vascular plexus in the synovial membrane, synovial fluid and blood vessels in the adjacent bone. Consequently, repair of damaged or worn articular cartilage is minimal. With increasing age the articular surface becomes increasingly undulated, developing minute ragged projections, probably due to wear and tear. Erosion may occur in 'dry' joints or where the viscosity of the synovial fluid is changed: in healthy joints articular cartilage changes are extremely slow.

Fibrous capsule

A fibrous capsule completely encloses the joint, forming a cuff with its margins attached continuously around the articular ends of the bones (Fig. 1.1), unless there are synovial outpouchings. It is perforated by nerves and blood vessels and has thickenings of parallel bundles of collagen, referred to as capsular thickenings. The joint capsule may be partly replaced by the tendons of adjacent muscles or their expansions. Accessory ligaments are separate from the capsule and may be either extracapsular or intracapsular.

The joint capsule and its associated thickenings, although yielding little to tension, are pliant and do not resist normal actions, but will resist excessive or abnormal movements.

Synovial membrane

Synovial membrane lines the fibrous capsule and covers all exposed bony surfaces and intracapsular structures (Fig. 1.1). In many joints fat pads occur in the synovial membrane, being flexible elastic cushions occupying potential spaces and irregularities within the joint which are not completely filled by synovial fluid. During movement these fat pads change shape. The synovial membrane is responsible for the production of synovial fluid, as well as removing debris from the joint space.

Synovial fluid

A clear viscous fluid found in synovial joints, bursae and tendon sheaths: its viscosity changing with the type of movement, loading conditions and joint temperature. Its volume is low, even in large joints such as the knee. Synovial fluid provides a liquid environment within the joint, and for the joint surfaces nutrition, lubrication and reduction of erosion.

Various models of lubrication have been proposed; however, given the variation in geometry, structure and activity at joints multiple modes of lubrication are likely to operate under different conditions at different joints.

The precise configuration of the surface, the degree of congruence and arrangement of the joint capsule and associated ligaments all influence the type and range of movement permitted at a joint.

CLASSIFICATION OF SYNOVIAL JOINTS

Most joints have two surfaces, the general shape of which is used to classify them into seven varieties.

Plane joints. The surfaces are flat or at least relatively flat and of a similar extent. The movement possible is a gliding or twisting of one surface against the other, usually within narrow limits.

Hinge (ginglymus) joints. The surfaces are arranged to permit movement in one direction only and usually have a high degree of congruence. They are supported by strong collateral ligaments.

Pivot (trochoid) joints. The bones are arranged so that one rotates within a fibro-osseous ring about a single axis.

Saddle (sellar) joints. The surfaces are reciprocally concavoconvex, with movement occurring about two mutually perpendicular axes. Occasionally there is a small degree of movement about a third axis.

Ball-and-socket (spheroidal) joints. The rounded 'head' of one bone fits into a socket of the other, permitting movement about three mutually perpendicular axes.

Condyloid joints. Modified form of ball-and-socket joint permitting active movement about two perpendicular axes; however, passive movement may occur about a third axis.

Ellipsoid joints. Another form of ball-and-socket joint having ellipsoid surfaces, with movement occurring about two perpendicular axes.

The analysis of changes in position of a joint can be determined by considering movement about three mutually perpendicular axes, usually corresponding with the cardinal planes of the body. When movement is limited to one axis the joint is termed uniaxial; it has one degree of freedom of movement. If independent movement can occur about two axes the joint is biaxial, with two degrees of freedom of movement. When independent movement can occur about three axes it is multiaxial and has three degrees of freedom of movement.

MOVEMENT AT ARTICULAR SURFACES

The movements occurring between articular surfaces are complex, being combinations of spin, roll and glide: rarely is movement at a joint of one type only. Spin is described as one surface spinning (rotating) against the other occurring about a central axis (Fig. 1.2). In rolling one surface rolls across the other so that new parts of both surfaces continually come into contact with each other (Fig. 1.2). Sliding occurs when one surface slides over the other such that new parts on one surface continually make contact with the same part on the other surface.

Movement of one body segment with respect to another rarely takes place in a single plane, it usually occurs in two or three planes simultaneously producing a complex pattern of movement. Nevertheless, it is convenient to consider movement about each of three defined axes separately (Fig. 1.2). Movement about a transverse axis occurring in a paramedian plane is termed flexion and extension: that about an anteroposterior axis occurring in a coronal plane is abduction and adduction; while that about a vertical axis occurring in a transverse plane is medial and lateral rotation.

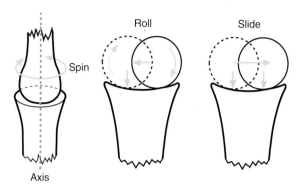

| **Fig 1.2** | Schematic representation of spin, roll and slide between articular surfaces. |

2 Flexibility and mobility

Determination of the range of movement at a joint, i.e. its flexibility, is influenced by a number of factors such as age, sex, and whether the movement is performed actively or passively. However, factors such as the activity in opposing muscle groups, the temperature of the surrounding environment and whether there has been a sufficient 'warm up' period will also influence the measured range of movement.

Flexibility tends to be joint-specific. It is not necessarily the case that because an individual exhibits great flexibility at one joint that all joints will be equally flexible. Although several studies have confirmed that in healthy subjects the range of movement is equivalent on the right and left side (Boone, 1979; Roaas and Andersson, 1982; Murray et al., 1985; Ahlberg et al., 1988; Svenningsen et al., 1989), it appears that the active range of movement responds to the habitual activity of that joint, especially when there has been trauma to the corresponding joint of the other limb (Poulis et al., 2000). This must be borne in mind when assessing range of movement and using the opposite joint as a reference, especially during rehabilitation.

AGE

Age can have a major influence on the range of movement at a joint, with younger individuals being more flexible than older individuals. Several investigators have reported on the ranges of movement in infants and young children (Watanabe et al., 1979; Waugh et al., 1983; Drews et al., 1984), with the effects being joint-specific and not influenced by sex. With increasing age range of movement decreases at most, if not all, joints. Consequently mean ranges of movement have been published for specific age groups (Boone, 1979; Walker et al., 1984; Downey et al., 1991) and should, where possible, be used as a standard against which measurement is evaluated. In the present text the changes in mean range of movement for specific joints is referred to; however, the tabulated required ranges for specific activities are not age-specific. They merely provide a guide as to the range of movement required to be able to perform a particular task or undertake particular activities.

The factors influencing these age-related ranges of movement include changes in activity level, muscle strength and neuromuscular coordination, degenerative disease and trauma, each of which will vary from individual to individual. In general, more physically active individuals tend to have greater ranges of movement than less active individuals.

SEX

Sex appears to be joint-specific; however, the differences between males and females is relatively small. No attempt has been made to identify these differences in this text; however, differences have been reported by Moll and Wright (1971), Beighton *et al.* (1973) and O'Driscoll and Thomenson (1982).

ACTIVE RANGE OF MOTION

This is the range of movement achieved during voluntary motion and provides information about coordination, muscle strength and the willingness to move: movement may be limited due to pain or the expectation of pain. The active range of motion tends to be less than that achieved passively.

PASSIVE RANGE OF MOTION

This is the range of movement achieved by an examiner without any contribution from the subject. It is normally greater than the active range of motion since each joint permits an additional amount of movement not under voluntary control. Testing the passive range of motion provides information about the integrity of the articular surfaces, as well as the extensibility of the soft tissues surrounding the joint.

FINAL RESISTANCE TO MOVEMENT

The final resistance to movement during passive testing may give an indication as to the factors restricting further motion. Normally the final resistance to movement will be: soft, due to soft tissue contact; firm, due to tension developed in the joint capsule, associated ligaments and muscles; or hard, due to bony contact. However, if the range of movement is prematurely arrested the final resistance to movement will still be either soft, firm or hard. If it is soft this may indicate soft tissue oedema or synovitis; if it is firm this indicates either soft tissue contracture or increased muscle tone; if it is hard this may indicate osteoarthritis, loose bodies within the joint space or a fracture. Occasionally there may be no final resistance because pain prevents little or no movement at the joint; such a situation may indicate joint inflammation, bursitis, an abscess, a fracture or a psychological problem.

3 Principles of measurement

Joint motion can be estimated visually; however, this provides no permanent objective record and makes comparisons between different assessment sessions difficult. The use of an objective method of measurement is necessary if the effectiveness of specific treatment regimens or rehabilitation programmes is to be evaluated. Therefore, some form of measuring device is required: these range from simple goniometers to sophisticated electromechanical devices, all of which have their advantages and disadvantages. In a clinical environment the simple goniometer may be the most appropriate, whereas in large-scale studies or those requiring more or less continuous measurement of joint position more sophisticated equipment will be more appropriate. Irrespective of the measuring device employed specific procedures must be followed to ensure correct alignment/positioning so that the movement of interest is being measured. Care must also be taken to ensure that the measurement being taken is valid and reliable.

Prior to undertaking measuring the relevant bony landmarks must be accurately identified and palpated, the examiner should be aware of the most appropriate position in which to place the subject, together with the stabilisation of body segments. In addition, the device must be correctly aligned with specific landmarks and the readings taken correctly. The determination of the range of movement for each joint considered in Section 2 is based on the use of a simple two-arm goniometer, the centre of which is placed over a specific bony landmark with the proximal and distal arms also aligned with particular landmarks. If using more sophisticated equipment the manufacturer's instructions must be strictly followed, with its limitations also being taken into account. The subsequent measurement of joint motion must be performed and recorded as accurately as possible, with movement being recorded as the maximum number of degrees a joint moves in a particular plane of motion.

VALIDITY AND RELIABILITY

To provide meaningful information measurements must be valid and reliable. Validity is the extent to which the device measures what it is supposed to measure, while reliability is the consistency between successive measurements of the same variable on the same subject under the same conditions.

Validity is often taken for granted without being specifically assessed. The assumption being that aligning a goniometer with specific landmarks and measuring the change in angle during movement represents the angular change at the joint. This takes no account of changing axes of motion or changes in the overlying soft tissues with respect to the underlying bony landmarks. The issue of validity has, however, led to the establishment of criterion-based validity for various types of goniometer in clinical applications, often based on comparisons with an accepted 'gold standard'. Nevertheless, in practice providing specific relevant landmarks have been identified the measurement is deemed valid.

A measurement is reliable if successive measurements under the same conditions give the same result. A highly reliable measurement has little measurement error; conversely a measurement with poor reliability contains a large amount of measurement error. A measurement with poor reliability cannot be depended upon and, therefore, should be avoided.

The measurement of range of motion is subject to several sources of error: changes in position of the axis of movement, variations in subject effort in active range of motion and variation in the force applied in passive range of motion. Not surprisingly measuring a fixed joint position is more reliable than measuring range of motion. Reliability also varies from joint to joint (Boone *et al.*, 1978), being higher for the limbs (Low, 1976; Hellebrandt *et al.*, 1985) than for the vertebral column (Fitzgerald *et al.*, 1983; Tucci *et al.*, 1986; Youdas *et al.*, 1991). In general, the more complex the joint the less reliable the measurement.

Reliability has also been observed to be higher when successive measurements are made by the same examiner (intratester reliability) rather than by different examiners (intertester reliability). Intertester reliability can, however, be improved when all examiners use consistent, well-defined test positions and measurement techniques. An additional factor influencing reliability is the time interval between successive measurements, with longer time intervals (days and weeks rather than hours) being less reliable.

To improve reliability Norkin and White (1995) recommend the following:

- Use consistent, well-defined test positions and landmarks
- The same amount of force should be applied to move the body segment in the assessment of the passive range of movement
- Subjects should be encouraged to exert the same effort to perform a movement in the assessment of the active range of movement
- Repeated measures should be taken with the same measuring device to reduce the variability of measurement

- Where possible successive measurements should be taken by the same examiner.

It has been suggested that there should be at least a 5° difference in joint motion before a true increase or decrease in the range of movement is accepted (Boone *et al.*, 1978).

4 Clinical application

Determining the alignment of joints and their ranges of movement are important adjuncts in assessing joint function, and are often undertaken as part of a more comprehensive assessment of the individual, which may also include the assessment of muscle strength and neurological, cardiovascular and respiratory function.

An assessment of joint alignment will indicate whether the pattern of forces transmitted across the joint is within acceptable limits or whether it will lead to degenerative changes and compromise function.

The assessment of the range of movement enables the presence or absence of dysfunction to be determined, a diagnosis to be made, treatment goals to be developed, progress during rehabilitation to be monitored, and orthoses to be prescribed. In addition it also provides the individual with the motivation to achieve a specific objective, particularly following trauma or a stroke.

Section 2

5 Pectoral girdle

INTRODUCTION

The pectoral girdle provides articulation of the upper limbs with the trunk; however, there is no direct articulation with the vertebral column. It articulates with the thoracic cage only, enabling forces generated in the upper limb to be partially transferred to the axial skeleton without restricting movement of the pectoral girdle or upper limb. The pectoral girdle consists of the scapula and clavicle on each side, with the scapula slung from the thoracic cage in muscle and the clavicle acting as a strut between the scapula and thorax. The clavicle articulates with the thorax by the sternoclavicular joint and with the scapula by the acromioclavicular joint. The clavicle moves with respect to the sternum, the scapula with respect to the clavicle and chest wall, and the humerus with respect to the scapula, thus providing the upper limb with its wide range of movement.

STERNOCLAVICULAR JOINT
Anatomy

The articulation is between the expanded medial end of the clavicle and the clavicular notch of the sternum, being a saddle-shaped synovial joint, i.e. the articular surfaces are reciprocally concavoconvex, although they do not have similar radii of curvatures and are therefore not completely congruent. The clavicular articular surface is larger than that on the sternum, which is set at 45° to the vertical, and projects above the upper margin of the sternum. The sternal surface is concave from above downwards and convex anteroposteriorly, while the clavicular surface is convex vertically and slightly concave horizontally, the concavity extending onto the inferior surface of the shaft for articulation with the first rib costal cartilage (Fig. 5.1). The clavicular surface overlaps the sternal surface both anteriorly and posteriorly.

The joint is surrounded by a strong fibrous capsule strengthened anteriorly, posteriorly and superiorly by anterior and posterior sternoclavicular ligaments and the interclavicular ligament respectively. Stability is primarily dependent on the strength of the joint capsule and associated ligaments, the costoclavicular ligament and the fibrocartilaginous intra-articular disc.

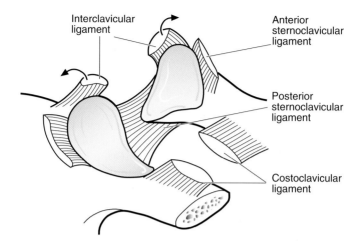

Interclavicular ligament

Anterior sternoclavicular ligament

Posterior sternoclavicular ligament

Costoclavicular ligament

Fig 5.1 The articular surfaces of the sternoclavicular joint: the capsule has been omitted.

Range of movement

Functionally the sternoclavicular joint is a ball-and-socket synovial joint permitting elevation/depression, protraction/retraction and axial rotation. Except for axial rotation the axes of movement are through the costoclavicular ligament and involve gliding between the clavicle and the intra-articular disc and between the disc and the sternum. Elevation/depression and protraction/retraction are both active movements, while axial rotation is passive, being produced by rotation of the scapula transmitted to the clavicle by the coracoclavicular ligament.

Elevation and depression

Movement occurs about an horizontal oblique axis passing anterolaterally through the costoclavicular ligament (Fig. 5.2a). Two separate axes have been proposed, one for the clavicle against the disc and one for the disc against the sternum (Ljunggren, 1979); nevertheless, functionally the combined axis passes through the costoclavicular ligament. Because the axis is not through the joint centre, as the lateral end of the clavicle moves in one direction the medial end moves in the opposite direction. Elevation of the lateral end of the clavicle produces a downward and lateral movement of the medial end: the reverse occurs with depression of the lateral end of the clavicle. The total angular range of movement is 60°, with elevation being the greater: in terms of linear displacement of the lateral end of the clavicle there is approximately 10 cm of elevation and 3 cm of depression. Elevation is limited by tension in the costoclavicular ligament and subclavius, depression by tension in the interclavicular ligament and intra-articular disc.

Protraction and retraction

Movement occurs about a vertical oblique axis running inferolaterally through the middle part of the costoclavicular ligament (Fig. 5.2b). Because the axis is not through the joint centre forward movement (protraction) of the lateral end of the clavicle produces a backward movement of the medial end: the reverse occurs in retraction. The total angular range of movement is 35°, with protraction being the greater: in terms of linear displacement the lateral end of the clavicle moves forward approximately 5 cm in protraction and backward 2 cm in retraction. Protraction is limited by tension in the anterior sternoclavicular and costoclavicular ligaments, and retraction by tension in the posterior sternoclavicular and costoclavicular ligaments.

Axial rotation

The axis of movement passes through the centres of the sternoclavicular and acromioclavicular joints (Fig. 5.2c). Axial rotation is possible due to the incongruence of the articular surfaces, the presence of the intra-articular disc, and the relative laxness of the capsular thickenings. The range of movement is between 20° and 40°, depending on the position of the clavicle, being least when the clavicle is in the frontal plane and increasing with retraction.

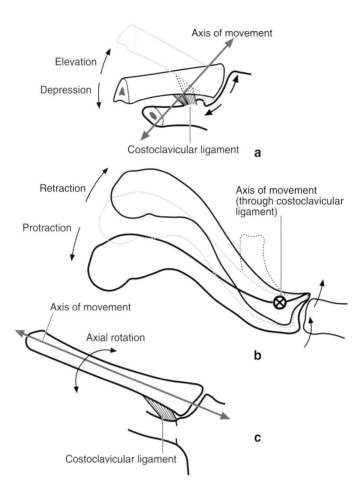

Fig 5.2 Movements of the clavicle at the sternoclavicular joint:
(a) elevation and depression; (b) protraction and retraction;
(c) axial rotation.

ACROMIOCLAVICULAR JOINT
Anatomy

The joint is a plane synovial joint being the articulation between an oval flat facet on the lateral end of the clavicle and a similar facet on the anteromedial border of the acromion process. The major axis of the joint runs from anterolateral to posteromedial, with the clavicular facet facing posterolaterally. A wedge-shaped fibrocartilaginous disc partially separates the articular surfaces from above.

A loose fibrous capsule surrounds the joint reinforced by capsular thickenings of variable thickness. Stability is essentially provided by the coracoclavicular ligament.

Range of movement

All movements at the joint are entirely passive, being produced by movements of the scapula; the movements, except axial rotation, are gliding of one articular surface against the other.

Movement about a vertical axis

Associated with protraction/retraction of the scapula the axis of movement passes vertically through the lateral end of the clavicle midway between the joint and the coracoclavicular ligament (Fig. 5.3a). As the acromion glides posteriorly with respect to the clavicle (retraction) the angle between them increases, while as the acromion glides anteriorly (protraction) the angle decreases (Fig. 5.3a). Posterior movement is limited by tension in the anterior joint capsule and coracoclavicular ligament (trapezoid part): anterior movement is limited by tension in the posterior joint capsule and coracoclavicular ligament (conoid part).

Movement about a sagittal axis

Associated with elevation/depression of the scapula the axis of movement passes through the joint centre (Fig. 5.3b). The total range of movement is 15°, with elevation limited by tension in the coracoclavicular ligament and depression by contact between the clavicle and coracoid process.

Axial rotation

Associated with medial and lateral rotation of the scapula, i.e. when the glenoid fossa faces inferiorly and superiorly respectively. The range of rotation of the scapula against the chest wall is 30° and occurs about an axis passing through the conoid part of the coracoclavicular ligament and

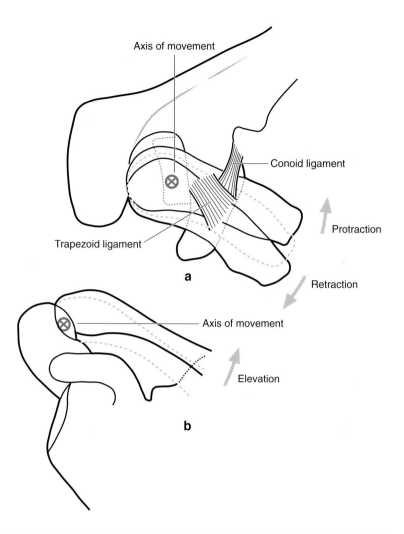

Axis of movement

Conoid ligament

Protraction

Trapezoid ligament

a

Retraction

Axis of movement

Elevation

b

Fig 5.3 Movement at the acromioclavicular joint: (a) about a vertical axis associated with protraction and retraction of the scapula; (b) about a parasagittal axis associated with elevation and depression of the scapula.

the acromioclavicular joint. Movement is limited by tension in the coracoclavicular ligament.

MOVEMENT OF THE PECTORAL GIRDLE AS A WHOLE

Movement of the pectoral girdle accompanies almost all movements of the shoulder joint, thereby increasing the range of movement of the upper limb.

Lateral and medial translation of the scapula

Lateral movement of the scapula around the chest wall brings it to lie more in a sagittal plane with the glenoid fossa facing more anteriorly (Fig. 5.4a, b). Movement towards the vertebral column brings the scapula to lie in a more frontal plane with the glenoid fossa facing more laterally. The two extremes of scapula movement form an angle of 40° to 45° (Fig. 5.4a), while the angle between the clavicle and scapula decreases to 60° with lateral movement and increases to 70° with medial movement (Fig. 5.4a). The total range of linear translation of the scapula around the chest wall is of the order of 15 cm.

Elevation and depression of the scapula

This has a linear range of 10–12 cm and is usually accompanied by rotation of the scapula so that the glenoid fossa comes to face more superiorly (Fig. 5.4c). Rotation of the scapula with respect to the chest wall occurs about an axis perpendicular to the plane of the scapula situated below the root of the spine of the scapula (Fig. 5.4d).

Rotation of the clavicle

During abduction or flexion of the upper limb the clavicle rotates about its long axis such that its superior surface faces increasingly posterior.

Movements of the pectoral girdle tend not to occur as pure movement, but involve some degree of each movement. Evaluation of the ranges of motion of the shoulder complex, i.e. the pectoral girdle and shoulder joint, are given in Chapter 6.

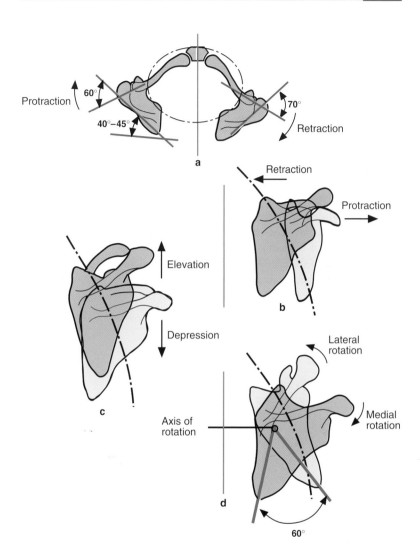

Fig 5.4 Movements of the pectoral girdle: protraction and retraction:
(a) viewed from above, (b) from behind; (c) elevation
and depression; (d) axial rotation.

6 Shoulder joint

ANATOMY

The shoulder joint is a synovial ball-and-socket joint between the head of the humerus and the glenoid fossa of the scapula. Only one-third of the humeral head is in contact with the glenoid fossa at any time for all joint positions: stability has been compromised at the expense of mobility.

In the frontal plane the axis of the head and neck forms an angle of 135° to 140° (angle of inclination) with the long axis of the shaft, so that the centre of the humeral head lies approximately 1 cm medial to the long axis. The axis of the head and neck is also retroverted 30° to 40° with respect to the shaft (Fig. 6.1); the degree of retroversion varies with age and race.

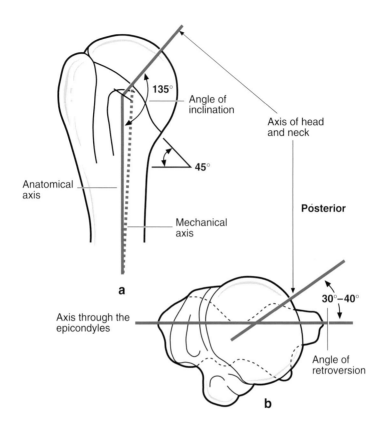

135°

Angle of inclination

Axis of head and neck

45°

Anatomical axis

Posterior

Mechanical axis

a

Axis through the epicondyles

30°–40°

Angle of retroversion

b

Fig 6.1 The articular surface of the humeral head also showing the associated angles of (a) inclination and (b) retroversion.

The head of the humerus forms two-fifths of a sphere and faces medially, superiorly and posteriorly with respect to the shaft. The pear-shaped glenoid fossa is a shallow socket at the superolateral angle of the scapula and faces laterally, anteriorly and slightly superiorly. The concavity is irregular and deepened by the glenoid labrum (Fig. 6.2).

The lax joint capsule attaches just outside the glenoid labrum proximally and to the anatomical neck distally medial to the lesser and greater tuberosities, except medially where it attaches to the shaft 1 cm below the articular margin. Although thick and strong anteriorly, where it is strengthened by glenohumeral ligaments, its laxity conveys little stability to the joint. The rotator cuff tendons (supraspinatus, infraspinatus, teres minor, subscapularis) blend with the capsule laterally and are important in maintaining joint integrity.

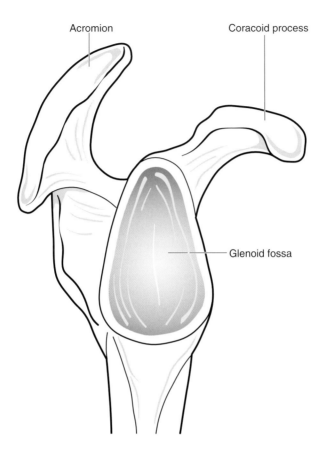

Acromion

Coracoid process

Glenoid fossa

Fig 6.2 The articular surface of the glenoid fossa of the scapula.

RANGES OF MOVEMENT

Movement is possible in all three planes; however, the axes about which movement occurs must be carefully defined as the plane of the scapula fossa is inclined approximately 45° to both the sagittal and coronal planes. Two sets of axes can, therefore, be defined; one with respect to the cardinal planes of the body and the other with respect to the plane of the scapula (Fig. 6.3): both sets of axes intersect at the centre of the humeral head. All movements, except axial rotation, are a combination of gliding and rolling of the articular surfaces against each other. When assessing the range of movement at the shoulder it is usually conducted with respect to the cardinal planes rather than to the plane of the scapula.

Even though the range of movement at the shoulder is relatively large, the mobility of the upper limb is increased by the mobility of the pectoral girdle. Except for the initial part of the movement flexion, extension, abduction and adduction are always accompanied by movement of the pectoral girdle. Shoulder movement is mainly concerned with bringing the arm to the horizontal position, while pectoral girdle movements (principally the scapula) enable the arm to move to the vertical. The association of shoulder and pectoral girdle movements increases the power and range of movement of the upper limb.

Flexion and extension

Movement of the arm about a transverse axis through the humeral head produces what is termed 'flexion' and 'extension'. When considered with respect to the plane of the scapula 'flexion' is a combination of flexion and abduction, while 'extension' is a combination of extension and adduction. The total range of active flexion and extension is approximately 230° (Boone and Azen, 1979), with flexion being greater (165°) than extension (65°). The range of both flexion and extension change with age. In neonates the passive range of flexion is 172° to 180° and of extension is 79° to 89°, decreasing to 169° and 69° respectively by age 5 (Watanabe *et al.*, 1979). The passive range of movement continues to decrease so that by age 60 flexion is 160° and extension 38° (Walker *et al.*, 1984).

Abduction and adduction

Movement of the arm about an anteroposterior axis through the humeral head produces what is termed 'abduction' and 'adduction'. With respect to the plane of the scapula 'abduction' is a combination of abduction and extension, while 'adduction' is a combination of adduction and flexion.

At all ages females tend to have a greater range of movement than males (Clarke *et al.*, 1975).

(a)

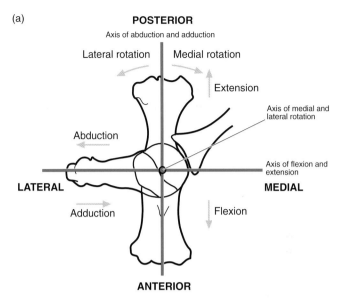

POSTERIOR

Axis of abduction and adduction

Lateral rotation | Medial rotation

Extension

Axis of medial and lateral rotation

Abduction

Axis of flexion and extension

LATERAL

MEDIAL

Adduction

Flexion

ANTERIOR

(b)

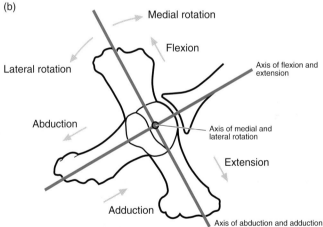

Medial rotation

Flexion

Lateral rotation

Axis of flexion and extension

Abduction

Axis of medial and lateral rotation

Extension

Adduction

Axis of abduction and adduction

Fig 6.3 The axes of movement at the shoulder joint: (a) with respect to the cardinal axes of the body; (b) with respect to the plane of the scapula.

Lateral and medial rotation

Rotation at the shoulder takes place about a longitudinal axis through the humerus between the centre of the head and centre of the capitulum. In lateral rotation the anterior surface of the arm faces laterally and in medial rotation it faces medially. The total range of rotation is of the order of 180° (AMA, 1988), with medial rotation being greater than 90° and lateral 80°. The combined range of rotation varies with the position of the arm, being greatest with the arm by the side, decreasing to 90° with the arm horizontal and negligible with the arm vertical. Rotation is limited by the extent of the articular surfaces, as well as tension in the joint capsule and muscles opposing movement. With increasing age the range of rotation decreases: in neonates lateral rotation is between 118° and 134°, with medial rotation 72° to 90° (Watanabe *et al.*, 1979), by age 5 the mean has reduced to 110° and 71° respectively with a gradual decrease with age, being 80° and 65° respectively age 60 and above (Downey *et al.*, 1991). At all ages females have greater rotation than males (Walker *et al.*, 1984).

The ranges of shoulder joint motion associated with some common activities are given in Table 6.1.

Table 6.1 Required range of shoulder joint movement (°) during common activities (adapted from Safaee-Rad *et al.*, 1990)

	Flexion	Abduction	Medial rotation
Eating	35	25	20
Drinking	45	35	25
Combing hair	110	100	45

EVALUATION OF RANGE OF MOTION

Evaluating the full range of motion at the shoulder requires free movement at the shoulder itself, as well as at the acromioclavicular and sternoclavicular joints: there also needs to be free movement of the scapula against the chest wall. Depending on the extent of stabilisation either shoulder joint motion or shoulder complex (all joints) motion can be determined.

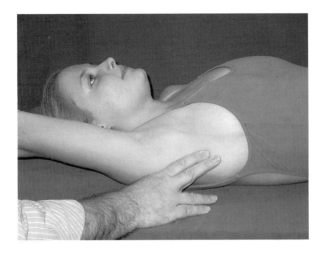

Fig 6.4 Determination of the range of flexion at the shoulder joint with the subject lying supine.

Flexion

With the subject lying supine, the knees flexed to flatten the lumbar spine, the shoulder in neutral abduction/adduction and rotation and the forearm in mid pronation/supination with the palm against the body, the scapula stabilised to prevent elevation, posterior tilting and upward rotation the arm is flexed (Fig. 6.4). To determine shoulder complex motion the thorax should also be stabilised to prevent extension of the spine. When determining shoulder joint motion the final resistance to movement is firm due to tension in the posterior band of the coracohumeral ligament, posterior joint capsule, teres minor, teres major and infraspinatus. For shoulder complex motion the final resistance to movement is also firm due to tension in latissimus dorsi and pectoralis major. To measure shoulder joint/shoulder complex flexion the centre of the goniometer is placed over the lateral aspect of the acromion process, with the proximal arm aligned along the midaxillary line and the distal arm in line with the lateral epicondyle of the humerus.

Extension

With the subject lying prone and the head turned away from the shoulder being tested, the shoulder in neutral abduction/adduction and rotation, the elbow in slight flexion and the forearm in mid pronation/supination with the palm facing the body, while the scapula is stabilised to prevent posterior elevation and anterior tilting of the scapula the arm is extended (Fig. 6.5). To determine shoulder complex motion the thorax should also be stabilised to prevent flexion of the spine. When measuring shoulder joint motion the final resistance to movement is firm due to tension in the anterior band of the coracohumeral ligament and anterior joint capsule. For shoulder complex movement the final resistance to movement is also firm due to tension in pectoralis major and serratus anterior. To measure shoulder joint/shoulder complex extension the centre of the goniometer is placed over the lateral aspect of the acromion process, with the proximal arm aligned with the midaxillary line and the distal arm in line with the lateral epicondyle of the humerus.

Abduction

With the subject lying supine, the shoulder in neutral flexion/extension and full lateral rotation with the palm facing anteriorly and the elbow extended, while the scapula is stabilised to prevent upward rotation and elevation the arm is abducted (Fig. 6.6). To determine shoulder complex motion the thorax should also be stabilised to prevent lateral flexion of the trunk. When measuring shoulder joint motion the final resistance to movement is firm due to tension in the middle and inferior glenohumeral ligaments, inferior joint capsule, latissimus dorsi and pectoralis major. For shoulder complex motion the final resistance to movement is also firm due to tension in rhomboid minor, rhomboid major, and the middle and inferior parts of trapezius. To measure shoulder joint/shoulder complex abduction the centre of the goniometer is placed over the anterior aspect of the acromion process, with the proximal arm parallel to the midline of the sternum and the distal arm aligned with the medial midline of the humerus.

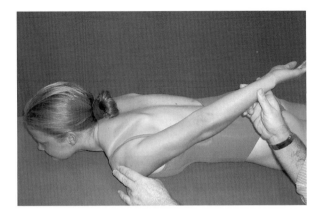

Fig 6.5 Determination of the range of extension at the shoulder joint with the subject lying prone.

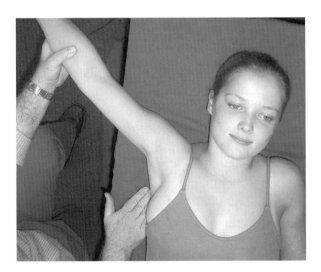

Fig 6.6 Determination of the range of abduction at the shoulder joint with the subject lying supine.

The measurement can also be taken with the subject sitting, standing (Fig. 6.7) or lying prone. When sitting or standing the centre of the goniometer is placed over the posterior aspect of the acromion process, with the proximal arm parallel to the vertebral spinous processes and the distal arm in line with the lateral epicondyle of the humerus.

Adduction

With the subject lying supine, the shoulder flexed sufficiently to allow the arm to pass in front of the chest and medially rotated 90° and the elbow extended, while the scapula is stabilised to prevent upward rotation and elevation, the arm is adducted across the front of the chest (Fig. 6.8). To determine shoulder complex motion the thorax should also be stabilised to prevent lateral flexion of the trunk. When measuring shoulder joint motion the final resistance to movement is firm due to tension in the superior glenohumeral ligament, superior joint capsule, and middle and posterior fibres of deltoid. For shoulder complex motion the final resistance to movement is also firm due to tension in the upper and middle parts of trapezius. To measure shoulder joint/shoulder complex adduction the centre of the goniometer is placed over the anterior aspect of the acromion process, with the proximal arm parallel to the midline of the sternum and the distal arm in line with the lateral epicondyle of the humerus.

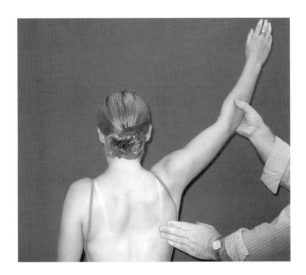

Fig 6.7 Determination of the range of abduction at the shoulder joint with the subject standing.

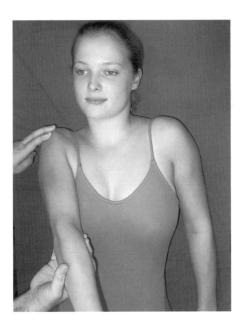

Fig 6.8 Determination of the range of adduction at the shoulder joint with the subject lying supine.

Alternatively, adduction can also be measured with the subject sitting or standing (Fig. 6.9), with stabilisation and goniometer placement the same as previously.

Lateral rotation

With the subject lying supine, the shoulder in 90° abduction, the elbow flexed 90° and the forearm pronated with the palm facing the feet, while the distal end of the humerus is stabilised, as well as the scapula towards the end of the movement to prevent posterior tilting, the arm is laterally rotated (Fig. 6.10). To determine shoulder complex motion the thorax should also be stabilised to prevent extension of the spine towards the end of the movement. When measuring shoulder joint motion the final resistance to movement is firm due to tension in the glenohumeral and coracohumeral ligaments, anterior joint capsule, subscapularis, pectoralis major, latissimus dorsi and teres major. For shoulder complex motion the final resistance to movement is also firm due to tension in serratus anterior and pectoralis minor. To measure shoulder joint/shoulder complex lateral rotation the centre of the goniometer is placed over the olecranon process, with the proximal arm either parallel or perpendicular to the supporting surface and the distal arm in line with the ulnar styloid process.

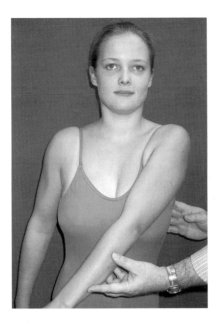

Fig 6.9 Determination of the range of adduction at the shoulder joint with the subject standing.

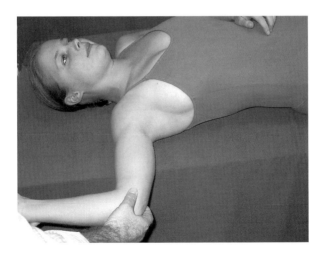

Fig 6.10 Determination of the range of lateral rotation at the shoulder joint with the subject lying supine and the shoulder abducted 90°.

Alternatively, lateral rotation can be determined with the subject sitting, standing or lying supine with the shoulder in neutral flexion/extension and abduction/adduction, the elbow flexed 90° and the forearm in mid pronation/supination, while the distal end of the humerus is stabilised the forearm is moved away from the midline (Fig. 6.11). To measure shoulder joint motion the centre of the goniometer is placed under the olecranon process, with the proximal arm aligned in the sagittal plane and the distal arm in line with the ulnar styloid process.

Medial rotation

With the subject lying supine, the shoulder in 90°, the elbow flexed and the forearm pronated with the palm facing the feet, while the distal end of the humerus is stabilised, as well as the scapula towards the end of the movement to prevent elevation and anterior tilting, the arm is medially rotated (Fig. 6.12). To determine shoulder complex motion the thorax is also stabilised to prevent flexion of the spine towards the end of the movement. When measuring shoulder joint motion the final resistance to movement is firm due to tension in the posterior joint capsule, infraspinatus and teres minor. For shoulder complex motion the final resistance to movement is also firm due to tension in rhomboid major, rhomboid minor and the middle and inferior parts of trapezius. To measure shoulder joint/shoulder complex medial rotation the centre of the goniometer is placed over the olecranon process, with the proximal arm either parallel or perpendicular to the supporting surface and the distal arm in line with the ulnar styloid process.

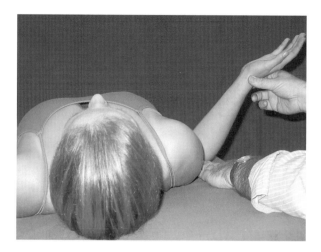

Fig 6.11 Determination of the range of lateral rotation at the shoulder joint with the subject lying supine and the shoulder in neutral.

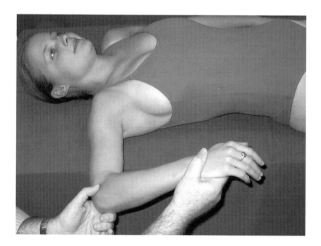

Fig 6.12 Determination of the range of medial rotation at the shoulder joint with the subject lying supine and the shoulder abducted 90°.

Alternatively, medial rotation can be determined with the subject sitting, standing or lying supine, the shoulder in neutral flexion/extension and abduction/adduction, the elbow flexed 90° and the forearm in mid pronation/supination, while the distal end of the humerus is stabilised the forearm is moved towards the midline (Fig. 6.13). To measure medial rotation of the shoulder complex the centre of the goniometer is placed under the olecranon process, with the proximal arm aligned in the sagittal plane and the distal arm in line with the ulnar styloid process.

A third method of assessing medial rotation is to determine the extent of the posterior reach. As well as shoulder movement it also requires movement at the elbow, wrist and thumb (Fig. 6.14). Posterior reach is defined as the highest segment of the back that can be reached by the thumb. Kronberg *et al.* (1990) reported that the thumb reaches the level of T4 and T5 in healthy young females and males respectively. The adult range is between T6 and T10.

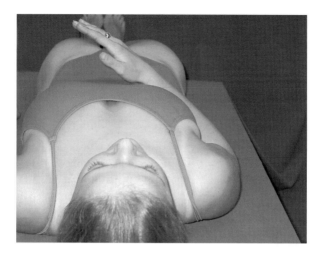

Fig 6.13 Determination of the range of medial rotation at the shoulder joint with the subject lying supine and the shoulder in neutral.

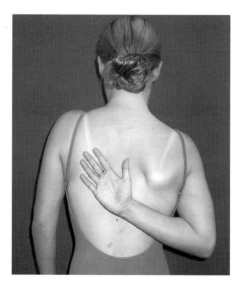

Fig 6.14 Medial rotation of the shoulder joint assessed by determining the extent of posterior reach: this method also requires movement at the elbow, wrist and thumb.

7 Elbow joint

ANATOMY

The elbow joint is the intermediate joint of the upper limb, being responsible for shortening and lengthening the upper limb as well as being subservient to the hand in that it enables the hand and fingers to be properly placed in space. It is a compound synovial hinge joint consisting of two distinct articulations, the humeroulnar and humeroradial joints.

The distal end of the humerus is expanded anteroinferiorly so that the trochlea lies anterior to the axis of the shaft (Fig. 7.1a). Similarly, the trochlear notch of the ulna projects anterosuperiorly lying anterior to the shaft of the ulna (Fig. 7.1a). This combined arrangement promotes a large range of flexion at the joint by delaying contact between the two bones. The long axes of the humerus and ulna coincide when viewed laterally, but deviate when viewed from the front forming the carrying angle (5–10° in males, 10–15° in females). The elbow joint axis runs from inferior, posterior and medial to superior, anterior and lateral, bisecting the carrying angle and passing through the middle of the trochlea (Fig. 7.1b).

The humeroulnar articulation is between the distal pulley-shaped trochlea of the humerus and the deep trochlear notch of the ulna. The trochlea almost forms a complete circle presenting an articular surface of 320–330°, the central groove being part of a spiral. The trochlear notch has a corresponding curved longitudinal ridge extending from the olecranon to the coronoid process: a transverse line crosses the notch at its deepest part. The obliquity of the notch to the shaft accounts for most of the carrying angle. The humeroradial articulation is between the distal rounded capitulum of the humerus and the shallow concave superior surface of the head of the radius, its raised margin articulating with the capitulotrochlear groove.

The joint capsule, which also encloses the superior radioulnar joint, generally attaches away from the articular margins superiorly and to the margins of the trochlear notch and annular ligament inferiorly: it has no direct attachment to the radius. It is strengthened at the sides by the medial and lateral collateral ligaments, being thinner and weaker anteriorly and posteriorly where it is reinforced by deep fibres from brachialis and triceps respectively.

Stability at the joint is partly determined by the shape of the articular surfaces, together with the collateral ligaments, and muscles crossing the

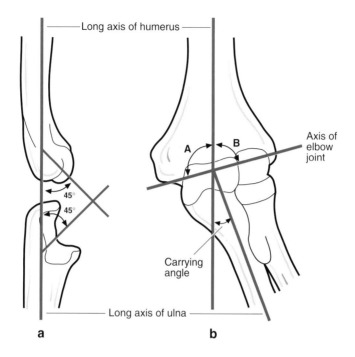

Fig 7.1 The distal end of the humerus and proximal ends of the radius and ulna: (a) the relation of the axes of the elbow joint; (b) the carrying angle.

joint, including the common tendons of the superficial flexors and extensors arising from the medial and lateral epicondyles of the humerus. In young children the radial head may dislocate through the annular ligament with traction forces applied to the forearm and/or hand.

RANGE OF MOVEMENT

Movement at the elbow joint is limited to flexion and extension in the sagittal plane about a transverse axis. Except at the extremes of flexion and extension movement between the humerus and radius and ulna is one of sliding, at the extremes it changes to rolling. During pronation/supination of the forearm there is a small degree of abduction/adduction respectively between the trochlear notch and trochlea. In addition, when fully extended some accessory abduction/adduction at the joint is possible when pressure is applied to the lower end of the forearm.

Flexion and extension

The total range of active flexion and extension is approximately 145° (Boone and Azen, 1979), being essentially accounted for by flexion; passive movement increases the range to 160° due to compression of the soft tissues of the arm and forearm. There may be a small amount (5°) of hyperextension, i.e. extension beyond the neutral joint position. In neonates the range of active flexion may be as large as 158° (Watanabe *et al.*, 1979), but decreases to 145° by age 5. It is not until age 60 that the range decreases slightly to 139° (Walker *et al.*, 1984), with older individuals also being unable to fully extend the elbow by approximately 6° (Walker *et al.*, 1984). There appears to be no difference in the range of flexion between males and females.

The range of elbow joint motion associated with some common activities is given in Table 7.1.

Table 7.1 Required range of flexion (°) at the elbow joint during some common activities (adapted from Safaee-Rad *et al.*, 1990)

	Flexion
Eating/drinking	130
Opening door	60
Reading	105
Using telephone	135
Rising from chair	95
Pouring from jug	60

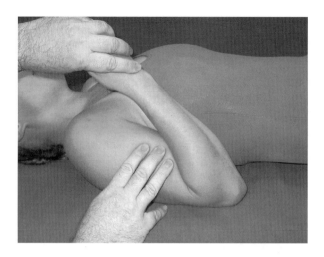

Fig 7.2 Determination of the range of flexion at the elbow joint with the subject lying supine.

EVALUATION OF RANGE OF MOTION
Flexion

With the subject lying supine, the shoulder in neutral flexion/extension and abduction/adduction and the forearm fully supinated with the palm facing upwards, while stabilising the distal end of the humerus the elbow is flexed (Fig. 7.2). The final resistance to movement is usually soft due to compression of the flexor muscles of the arm and forearm: if there is muscle atrophy the final resistance to movement may be hard due to contact between the coronoid process and coronoid fossa, and the head of the radius and radial fossa. If there is tension in the posterior capsule and triceps movement is arrested before contact between the arm and forearm, in which case the final resistance to movement is firm. To measure elbow flexion the centre of the goniometer is placed over the lateral epicondyle of the humerus, with the proximal arm aligned with the centre of the lateral aspect of the acromion process and the distal arm in line with the radial styloid process.

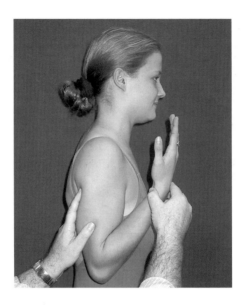

Fig 7.3 Determination of the range of flexion at the elbow joint with the subject standing.

Alternatively, flexion can be determined with the subject sitting or standing (Fig. 7.3).

Extension

With the subject lying supine and a pad under the distal end of the humerus, the shoulder in neutral flexion/extension and abduction/adduction and the forearm fully supinated, while stabilising the distal end of the humerus the elbow is extended (Fig. 7.4). The final resistance to movement is usually hard due to contact between the olecranon and olecranon fossa. If there is tension in the anterior capsule, collateral ligaments, biceps and brachialis the final resistance to movement is firm. To measure elbow extension the centre of the goniometer is placed over the lateral epicondyle of the humerus, with the proximal arm aligned with the centre of the lateral aspect of the acromion process and the distal arm in line with the radial styloid process.

Alternatively, extension can be determined with the subject sitting or standing (Fig. 7.5).

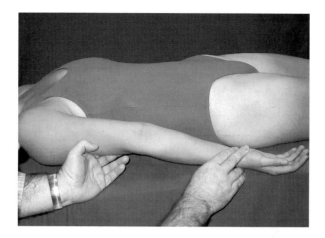

Fig 7.4   Determination of the range of extension at the elbow joint with the subject lying supine.

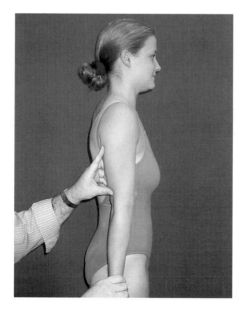

Fig 7.5   Determination of the range of extension at the elbow joint with the subject standing.

8 Superior and inferior radioulnar joints

ANATOMY

The radius and ulna articulate with each other at their proximal and distal ends by synovial joints and along their length by an interosseous membrane, permitting rotation around the ulna as in supination (bones crossing each other) and pronation (bones parallel to each other). In supination/pronation the hand is carried with the forearm rotation effectively giving an additional axis of movement at the wrist: functionally the hand articulates with the forearm via a ball-and-socket synovial joint.

Superior radioulnar joint

The articulation is between the bevelled circumference of the slightly oval radial head and the concave radial notch of the ulna and fibrous cartilage-lined annular ligament, which is narrower inferiorly to prevent downward displacement of the radial head (Fig. 8.1). Superiorly the radial collateral ligament fuses with the annular ligament, while it blends with the fibrous capsule of the elbow joint anteriorly and posteriorly. The joint is continuous with the elbow joint sharing the same joint capsule.

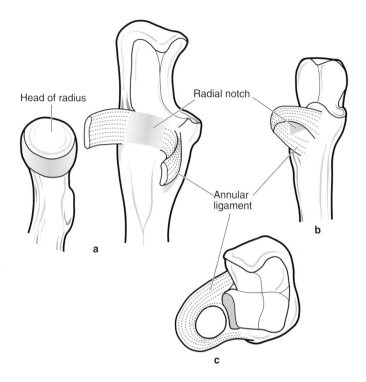

Head of radius

Radial notch

Annular ligament

a

b

c

Fig 8.1 The articular surfaces of the superior radioulnar joint: (a) with the surfaces exposed; (b) viewed from the front; (c) viewed from above.

The joint is inherently stable; however, the head of the radius may be pulled from the confines of the annular ligament in traction dislocation in children. During movement at the joint the head of the radius (a) rotates within the annular fibro-osseous ring; (b) rotates against the capitulum of the humerus; (c) is displaced slightly laterally; and (d) becomes tilted infero-laterally during pronation (Fig. 8.2).

The head of the radius can be palpated posteriorly in the depression on the posterolateral aspect of the elbow and can be felt moving during pronation and supination.

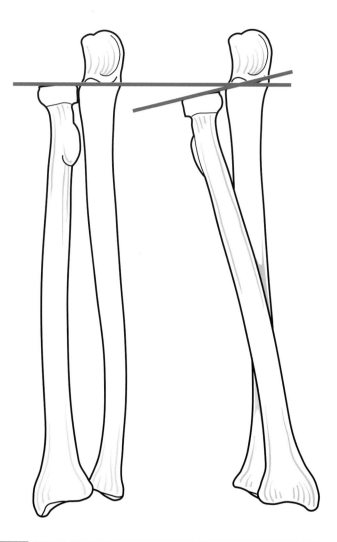

Fig 8.2   Movement of the radius at the superior radioulnar joint during pronation.

Inferior radioulnar joint

The articulation is between the slightly expanded head of the ulna and the concave ulnar notch of the radius (Fig. 8.3). The distal aspect of the ulnar head articulating with a triangular disc separating the inferior radioulnar joint from the radiocarpal joint: the disc is the principal structure uniting the two bones inferiorly.

A relatively weak loose fibrous capsule surrounds the joint attaching to the margins of the ulnar notch and corresponding regions of the ulnar head blending inferiorly with the anterior and posterior margins of the articular disc. The synovial membrane extends superiorly anterior to the interosseous membrane forming the recessus sacciformis.

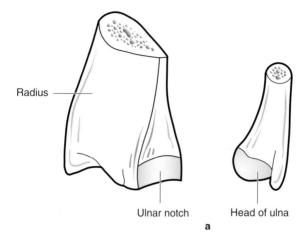

Radius

Ulnar notch   Head of ulna

a

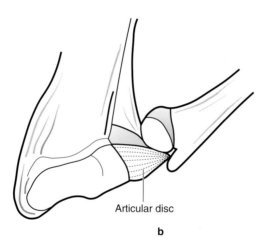

Articular disc

b

Fig 8.3   The articular surfaces of the inferior radioulnar joint: (a) without the articular disc; (b) with the disc in situ.

Stability is provided by the articular disc, interosseous membrane and pronator quadratus. During pronation the distal end of the radius rotates around the head of the ulna, however because the axis of pronation/supination coincides with the axis of the hand (3rd metacarpal) radial rotation is accompanied by slight extension and lateral displacement of the ulna inferiorly (Fig. 8.4). This lateral displacement of the ulna is permitted by medial displacement of the ulna at the elbow between the trochlea of the humerus and the trochlear notch of the ulna.

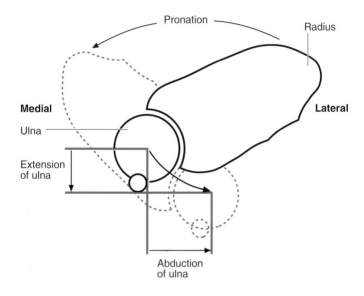

Fig 8.4   Movement of the radius and ulna at the inferior radioulnar joint during pronation.

RANGE OF MOVEMENT

Movement at the radioulnar joints is pronation and supination, being rotation of the radius about the ulna at both joints. Accessory movements are possible at both joints: superiorly the head of the radius can be moved anteroposteriorly with respect to both the ulna and capitulum, while inferiorly the head of the ulna can be moved anteroposteriorly with respect to the radius.

Pronation and supination

The total range of pronation and supination in neonates may be as large as 190°, being approximately 95° each (Watanabe *et al.*, 1979). With increasing age the range decreases to 68° pronation and 83° supination at age 60 (Walker *et al.*, 1984).

The range of pronation/supination associated with some common activities is given in Table 8.1.

Table 8.1 Required range of pronation and supination (°) of the forearm during some common activities (adapted from Morrey *et al.*, 1981)

	Pronation	Supination
Eating	45	
Opening door	35	25
Reading	50	
Using telephone	40	25
Rising from chair	35	
Pouring from jug	45	25

Evaluation of range of motion

Pronation

With the subject sitting, the shoulder in neutral flexion/extension, abduction/adduction and rotation, the elbow flexed 90° and the forearm supported in the mid pronated/supinated position so that the thumb points upwards, with the distal end of the humerus stabilised the forearm is pronated (Fig. 8.5). The final resistance to movement is firm due to tension in the posterior radioulnar ligament, interosseous membrane, supinator and biceps: if there is contact between the radius and ulna the final resistance to movement will be hard. To measure pronation the centre of the goniometer is placed lateral to the ulnar styloid process, with the proximal arm parallel to the anterior midline of the humerus and the distal arm across the posterior aspect of the forearm just proximal to the radial and ulnar styloid processes.

Supination

With the subject sitting, the shoulder in neutral flexion/extension, abduction/adduction and rotation, the elbow flexed 90° and the forearm supported in the mid pronated/supinated position so that the thumb points upwards, with the distal end of the humerus stabilised the forearm is supinated (Fig. 8.6). The final resistance to movement is firm due to tension in the anterior radioulnar ligament, interosseous membrane, oblique cord, pronator teres and pronator quadratus. To measure supination the centre of the goniometer is placed medial to the ulnar styloid process, with the proximal arm parallel to the anterior midline of the humerus and the distal arm across the anterior aspect of the forearm just proximal to the radial and ulnar styloid processes.

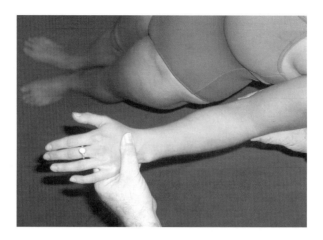

Fig 8.5   Determination of the range of pronation of the forearm.

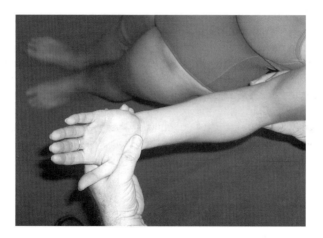

Fig 8.6   Determination of the range of supination of the forearm.

9 Wrist joint

INTRODUCTION

The wrist comprises a series of articulations between the carpal bones (intercarpal joints) and the articulation with the forearm (radiocarpal joint). Functionally the carpal bones are arranged and move as two rows of four bones, the proximal row being from lateral to medial the scaphoid, lunate, triquetral and pisiform, and the distal row the trapezium, trapezoid, capitate and hamate; the joint between the two rows being the midcarpal joint. The functional interdependence of the wrist and hand means that movements at both the radiocarpal and midcarpal joints accompany all movements of the hand. Movements possible are flexion/extension in a sagittal plane about a mediolateral axis and abduction/adduction in the frontal plane about an anteroposterior axis: both axes passing through the head of the capitate (Youm and Yoon, 1979).

Each row of carpal bones form a transverse arch concave anteriorly, being partly maintained by the flexor retinaculum, which attaches medially to the pisiform and hook of hamate and laterally to the scaphoid tubercle and both lips of the groove on the trapezium (Fig. 9.1).

ANATOMY
Radiocarpal joint

The radiocarpal joint is an ellipsoid synovial joint allowing movement in two directions. The articulation is between the distal end of the radius and the articular disc, which form a continuous concave ellipsoid surface shallower transversely than anteroposteriorly, and the almost continuous convex articular surface of the proximal row of carpal bones (Fig. 9.2). In the neutral position the scaphoid lies opposite the lateral triangular area of the radius, the lunate opposite the medial quadrangular area and articular disc and the triquetral opposite the medial part of the disc and against the medial joint capsule.

A fibrous capsule completely encloses the joint passing from the distal margins of the radius and ulna to the proximal carpal row. It is thickened anteriorly and posteriorly and blends at the sides with radial and ulnar collateral ligaments. The joint is relatively stable due to the attachment of the flexor retinaculum and the many tendons crossing anteriorly and posteriorly into the hand.

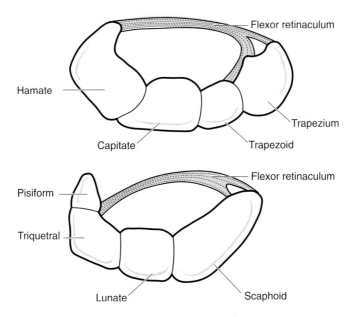

Fig 9.1 Arrangement of the carpal bones showing the attachment of the flexor retinaculum to form the carpal tunnel.

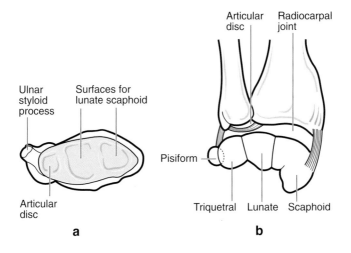

Fig 9.2 The articular surfaces of the wrist joint: (a) the radius and intra-articular disc; (b) the proximal row of carpal bones.

Midcarpal joint

The midcarpal joint is the articulation between the adjacent surfaces of the proximal and distal row of carpal bones: laterally it consists of two plane surfaces with a slight distal convexity, while the larger medial part is concave distally (Fig. 9.3). Laterally the trapezium and trapezoid articulate with the scaphoid, the capitate with the scaphoid and lunate centrally, and the hamate with the lunate and triquetral medially.

The joint is surrounded by a fibrous capsule of irregular bands passing between the two rows, being strengthened at the sides by the radial and ulnar collateral ligaments. The joint is relatively stable due to the attachment of the flexor retinaculum and the many tendons crossing anteriorly and posteriorly into the hand.

RANGE OF MOVEMENT

Although the radiocarpal and midcarpal joints each permit flexion/extension and abduction/adduction, movement occurs simultaneously at both joints about single axes, which pass through the head of the capitate. The contribution of each joint to each movement differs due to the anatomy of the individual joints. Accessory anteroposterior movements are possible at both joints if either the radius and ulna or proximal row of carpal bones are stabilised. Applying a longitudinal force separates the proximal row of carpal bones from the radius and articular disc, and the joint surfaces of the proximal and distal rows.

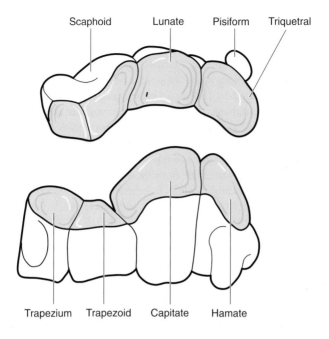

Scaphoid   Lunate   Pisiform   Triquetral

Trapezium   Trapezoid   Capitate   Hamate

Fig 9.3 The articular surfaces of the midcarpal joint.

Flexion and extension

In flexion the palm of the hand moves anteriorly approaching the anterior surface of the forearm, while in extension the dorsum of the hand moves posteriorly to approach the posterior surface of the forearm. The total range of movement is in excess of 180° in neonates, being up to to 96° flexion and 89° extension (Watanabe *et al.*, 1979), however by late teens these values have decreased to 75° and 73° respectively (Boone, 1979). With increasing age the range of flexion and extension continue to decrease so that by the seventh decade it is 62° flexion and 61° extension (Walker *et al.*, 1984). At all ages females tend to have a greater range of motion than males.

Flexion at the radiocarpal joint is freer than extension, while extension at the midcarpal joint is freer than flexion. During flexion the scaphoid and lunate move within the concave distal surface of the radius so that their proximal surfaces face posterosuperiorly: the scaphoid also twists about its long axis so that its tubercle is less prominent. At the same time the head of the capitate rotates within the concavity formed by the scaphoid and lunate, while the hamate rotates against the triquetral. During extension the twisting of the scaphoid about its long axis makes its tubercle more prominent.

The range of flexion and extension associated with some common activities are given in Table 9.1.

Table 9.1 Required range of movement (°) at the wrist during common activities (adapted from Brumfield and Champoux, 1984)

	Flexion	Extension	Abduction	Adduction
Eating/drinking	5	40		
Reading		35		
Writing		15		10
Using telephone		45	15	
Rising from chair		65	15	
Pouring from jug	10	30	10	
Placing hand on:				
Neck	5			10
Waist	15			
Chest	20			
Back of head		15		
Shoe		15		

Abduction and adduction

Abduction and adduction, also referred to as radial and ulnar deviation, is movement of the hand such that the fingers move away from or towards the midline respectively. At all ages the range of adduction exceeds that of abduction and is generally greater in females than in males. In young children the range of abduction is 24° and of adduction is 39°, decreasing to 20° and 36° respectively by age 20 (Boone, 1979). Further decreases with increasing age result in a range of 20° abduction and 28° adduction at age 60 (Walker *et al.*, 1984).

At both the radiocarpal and midcarpal joints abduction is more limited than adduction. During abduction the triquetral moves medially to become clear of the radius, the lunate follows with the scaphoid tubercle approaching the radial styloid process. At the same time the capitate moves close to the triquetral separating the hamate from the lunate. During adduction the scaphoid rotates so that its tubercle moves away from the radial styloid process, the lunate moves entirely distal to the radius and the triquetral distal to the articular disc. At the same time the capitate rotates so that its distal part moves medially, the hamate separates from the triquetral and approaches the lunate.

Abduction/adduction at the midcarpal joint is accompanied by a twisting of the two rows of bones. In abduction the distal row twists in the direction of supination and extension, while the proximal row twists in the direction of pronation and flexion. A reverse twisting occurs in adduction.

The range of abduction and adduction associated with some common activities are given in Table 9.1.

EVALUATION OF THE RANGE OF MOTION
Flexion

With the subject sitting, the shoulder abducted 90° and the elbow flexed 90°, the forearm in mid pronation/supination with the palm facing inferiorly the forearm is supported and the hand free to move, with the radius and ulna stabilised the wrist is flexed while preventing abduction/adduction (Fig. 9.4). The final resistance to movement is firm due to tension in the dorsal intercarpal ligament and posterior joint capsule: if the fingers are flexed the range of movement is reduced due to tension in extensor digitorum, extensor indicis and extensor digiti minimi. To measure flexion the centre of the goniometer is placed over the medial aspect of the wrist distal to the ulnar styloid process, with the proximal arm aligned with a line joining the ulnar styloid and olecranon processes and the distal arm along the 5th metacarpal.

Alternatively, with the forearm supinated (Fig. 9.5) the centre of the goniometer is placed over the middle of the posterior aspect of the wrist, with the proximal arm along the posterior midline of the forearm and the distal arm along the 3rd metacarpal.

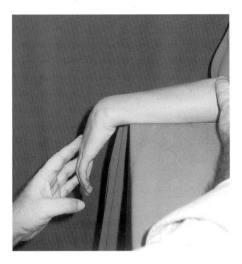

Fig 9.4 Determination of the range of flexion at the wrist with the subject seated and the forearm in mid pronation/supination.

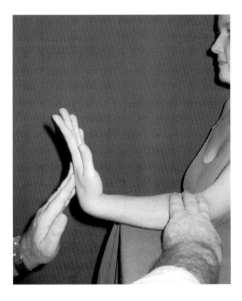

Fig 9.5 Determination of the range of flexion at the wrist with the subject seated and the forearm supinated.

Extension

With the subject sitting, the shoulder abducted 90° and the elbow flexed 90°, the forearm in mid pronation/supination with the palm facing inferiorly the forearm is supported and the hand free to move, with the radius and ulna stabilised the wrist is extended while preventing abduction/adduction (Fig. 9.6). The final resistance to movement is firm due to tension in the palmar intercarpal ligament and anterior joint capsule: if the fingers are flexed the range of movement is reduced due to tension in flexor digitorum superficialis and flexor digitorum profundus. The final resistance to movement may, however, be hard due to contact between the scaphoid and lunate and the radius. To measure extension the centre of the goniometer is placed over the medial aspect of the wrist distal to the ulnar styloid process, with the proximal arm aligned with a line joining the ulnar styloid and olecranon processes and the distal arm along the 5th metacarpal.

Alternatively, with the forearm supinated (Fig. 9.7) the centre of the goniometer is placed over the middle of the posterior aspect of the wrist, with the proximal arm along the posterior midline of the forearm and the distal arm along the 3rd metacarpal.

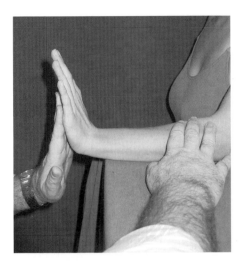

Fig 9.6 Determination of the range of extension at the wrist with the subject seated and the forearm in mid pronation/supination.

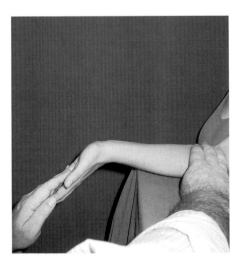

Fig 9.7 Determination of the range of extension at the wrist with the subject seated and the forearm supinated.

Abduction

With the subject sitting, the shoulder abducted 90° and the elbow flexed 90°, the forearm in mid pronation/supination with the palm facing inferiorly the forearm is supported and the hand free to move, with the radius, ulna and elbow joint stabilised the wrist is abducted (Fig. 9.8). The final resistance to movement is usually hard due to contact between the scaphoid and radial styloid process; however, it may be firm due to tension in the ulnar collateral and ulnar collateral carpal ligaments and medial part of the joint capsule. To measure abduction the centre of the goniometer is placed over the middle of the posterior aspect of the wrist (over the capitate), with the proximal arm along the posterior midline of the forearm and the distal arm along the 3rd metacarpal.

Adduction

With the subject sitting, the shoulder abducted 90° and the elbow flexed 90°, the forearm in mid pronation/supination with the palm facing inferiorly the forearm is supported and the hand free to move, with the radius, ulna and elbow joint stabilised the wrist is adducted (Fig. 9.9). The final resistance to movement is firm due to tension in the radial collateral and radial collateral carpal ligaments and lateral part of the joint capsule. To measure adduction the centre of the goniometer is placed over the middle of the posterior aspect of the wrist (over the capitate), with the proximal arm along the posterior midline of the forearm and the distal arm along the 3rd metacarpal.

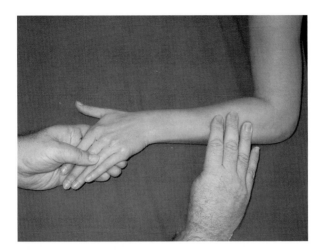

Fig 9.8 Determination of the range of abduction at the wrist with the subject seated and the forearm in mid pronation/supination.

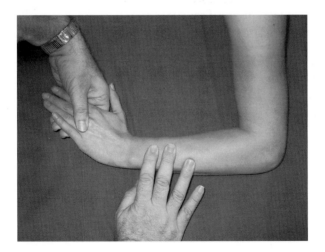

Fig 9.9 Determination of the range of adduction at the wrist with the subject seated and the forearm in mid pronation/supination.

10 Joints of the hand

INTRODUCTION

The hand consists of a series of joints arranged along individual rays (digits), which subserve the primary function of manipulation and gripping. The bases of the metacarpals articulate with the carpus via carpometacarpal joints, with the 1st carpometacarpal joint being extremely mobile and the common carpometacarpal joint permitting little movement. The heads of each metacarpal articulate with a proximal phalanx at the metacarpophalangeal joint, while adjacent phalanges articulate via interphalangeal joints. The axis of the hand runs along the middle finger (3rd digit), being in line with the long axis of the forearm.

THUMB
Introduction

The thumb is rotated approximately 90° with respect to the remaining digits, thus its movements will be in a different plane to those of the other digits. It is an extremely mobile and specialised digit, both of which are important prerequisites for the prehensile functioning of the hand.

First carpometacarpal joint
Anatomy

The articulation is between the base of the 1st metacarpal and the trapezium, being a saddle-shaped synovial joint; i.e. the articular surfaces are concavoconvex. The metacarpal is convex anteroposteriorly and concave perpendicular to this: the trapezium has reciprocal curvatures (Fig. 10.1). Because the tendons of the muscles producing movement lie parallel to the metacarpal the joint surfaces tend to grind against each other rather than roll or glide during movement.

The joint is surrounded by a strong but lax fibrous capsule thickened laterally by the radial carpometacarpal ligament, and anteriorly and posteriorly by anterior and posterior oblique ligaments. Stability is provided principally by the tendons crossing the joint.

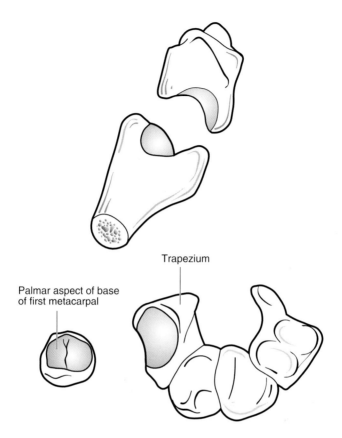

Trapezium

Palmar aspect of base
of first metacarpal

Fig 10.1   The articular surfaces of the carpometacarpal joint of the thumb.

Range of movement

Due to the shape of the articular surfaces and looseness of the joint
capsule the joint has a large degree of mobility, being flexion/extension,
abduction/adduction and axial rotation (opposition): flexion/extension and
abduction/adduction are in the plane of the palm and perpendicular to the
palm respectively.

Flexion and extension

The axis about which movement occurs passes through the base of the
metacarpal at the centres of curvature of the concave trapezium and convex metacarpal, running obliquely from posterior, lateral and proximal to

anterior, medial and distal. The total range of flexion and extension is 50°, towards the end of flexion the metacarpal rotates medially, while towards the end of extension it rotates laterally.

Abduction and adduction

The axis about which movement occurs passes through the trapezium at the centres of curvature of the concave metacarpal and the convex trapezium, running obliquely from medial, posterior and distal to lateral, anterior and proximal. The range of abduction is 70° (AAOS, 1994), adduction being the return of the thumb so that it lies in the plane of the palm.

Axial rotation

During opposition of the thumb medial rotation is initially passive due to the combined movements of flexion and abduction; however, when opponens pollicis contracts the rotation becomes active. Axial rotation is of the order of 40°.

Accessory movements

Accessory movements at the carpometacarpal joint can be produced by gripping the trapezium and metacarpal whereby the metacarpal can be moved both anteroposteriorly and mediolaterally, as well as producing distraction at the joint.

Evaluation of the range of motion

Flexion

With the subject sitting, the forearm supinated and resting on a supported surface, the wrist in neutral flexion/extension and abduction/adduction, the carpometacarpal joint in neutral abduction/adduction, the metacarpophalangeal and interphalangeal joints in neutral flexion/extension and the carpus stabilised with the hand resting on a supporting surface the carpometacarpal joint is flexed (Fig. 10.2). The final resistance to movement is usually soft due to compression of the thenar eminence against the palm of the hand; however, it may be firm due to tension in the posterior joint capsule, extensor pollicis brevis and abductor pollicis brevis. To measure flexion the centre of the goniometer is placed over the palmar aspect of the carpometacarpal joint, with the proximal arm along a line joining the radial styloid process and radial head and the distal arm along the anterior midline of the 1st metacarpal. The initial goniometer reading may not be 0°; however, the difference between the initial and final readings gives the range.

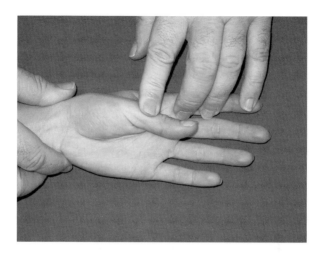

Fig 10.2   Determination of the range of flexion at the carpometacarpal joint of the thumb.

Extension

With the subject sitting, the forearm supinated and resting on a supported surface, the wrist in neutral flexion/extension and abduction/adduction, the carpometacarpal joint in neutral abduction/adduction, the metacarpophalangeal and interphalangeal joints in neutral flexion/extension and the carpus stabilised with the hand resting on a supporting surface the carpometacarpal joint is extended (Fig. 10.3). The final resistance to movement is firm due to tension in the anterior joint capsule, flexor pollicis brevis, adductor pollicis, opponens pollicis and the 1st dorsal interosseous. To measure extension the centre of the goniometer is placed over the palmar aspect of the carpometacarpal joint, with the proximal arm along a line joining the radial styloid process and radial head and the distal arm along the anterior midline of the 1st metacarpal. The initial goniometer reading may not be 0°; however, the difference between the initial and final readings gives the range.

Abduction

With the subject sitting, the forearm mid pronated/supinated and resting on a supporting surface, the wrist in neutral flexion/extension and abduction/adduction, the carpometacarpal, metacarpophalangeal and interphalangeal joints in neutral flexion/extension, and the carpus and 2nd metacarpal stabilised with the hand resting on a supporting surface the carpometacarpal joint is abducted (Fig. 10.4). The final resistance to movement is firm due to tension primarily in the fascia and skin of the web space between the thumb and index finger: there may also be tension in adductor pollicis and the 1st dorsal interosseous. To measure abduction the centre of the goniometer is placed over the lateral aspect of the radial styloid process, with the proximal arm in line with the midline of the 2nd metacarpal and the distal arm in line with the 1st metacarpal.

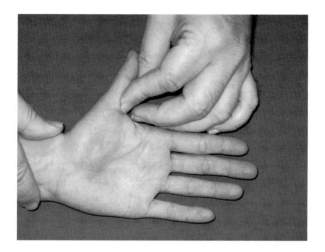

Fig 10.3 Determination of the range of extension at the carpometacarpal joint of the thumb.

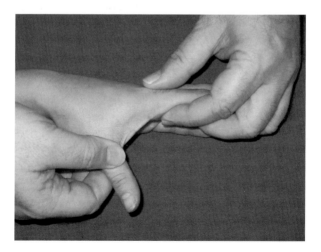

Fig 10.4 Determination of the range of abduction at the carpometacarpal joint of the thumb.

Metacarpophalangeal joint
Anatomy

A condyloid synovial joint between the rounded convex head of the metacarpal and the shallow oval concavity of the proximal phalanx (Fig. 10.5). The metacarpal head is wider anteriorly than posteriorly and has a greater curvature transversely than anteroposteriorly. The base of the proximal phalanx has a smaller articular surface than the metacarpal head, being increased by the fibrocartilaginous palmar ligament attached to its anterior surface.

It is surrounded by a loose fibrous capsule strengthened posteriorly by an expansion of extensor pollicis longus and at the sides by collateral ligaments. Stability is maintained by the collateral ligaments, flexor pollicis longus, extensor pollicis longus, extensor pollicis brevis, flexor pollicis brevis and abductor pollicis brevis.

Range of movement

The shape of the joint permits active movement in two planes, flexion/extension in the frontal plane and abduction/adduction in the sagittal plane, as well as passive axial rotation accompanying simultaneous flexion and abduction or when pressing the thumb against the index finger. Active axial rotation is always medially directed, while passive axial rotation can be in either direction.

Flexion and extension

Occurs about a single fixed transverse axis through the head of the metacarpal nine-tenths of its length from the base (Youm *et al.*, 1978). The range of flexion is 60° (AMA, 1988) and extension 0° under normal circumstances; however, it may be possible to extend the joint beyond the neutral position (hyperextension).

Abduction and adduction

Abduction is of the order of 15°, with adduction being negligible. The axis about which movement occurs passes anteroposteriorly through the metacarpal head.

Accessory movement

An accessory anteroposterior gliding of the proximal phalanx against the metacarpal can be elicited.

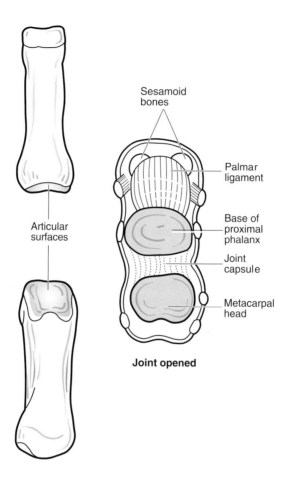

Sesamoid bones

Palmar ligament

Base of proximal phalanx

Joint capsule

Metacarpal head

Articular surfaces

Joint opened

Fig 10.5 The articular surfaces of the metacarpophalangeal joint of the thumb.

Evaluation of the range of motion

Flexion

With the subject sitting, the forearm supinated and resting on a supporting surface, the wrist and carpometacarpal joints in neutral flexion/extension and abduction/adduction, the interphalangeal joint in neutral flexion/extension and the 1st metacarpal stabilised with the hand resting on a supporting surface the metacarpophalangeal joint is flexed (Fig. 10.6). The final resistance to movement is usually firm due to tension in the posterior joint capsule, the collateral ligaments and extensor pollicis brevis; however, it may be hard due to contact between the palmar aspect of the proximal phalanx and the 1st metacarpal. To measure flexion the centre of the goniometer is placed over the posterior aspect of the joint, with the proximal arm in line with the metacarpal and the distal arm in line with the proximal phalanx.

Extension

With the subject sitting, the forearm supinated and resting on a supporting surface, the wrist and carpometacarpal joints in neutral flexion/extension and abduction/adduction, the interphalangeal joint in neutral flexion/extension and the 1st metacarpal stabilised with the hand resting on a supporting surface the metacarpophalangeal joint is extended (Fig. 10.7). The final resistance to movement is firm due to tension in the anterior joint capsule, the palmar ligament and flexor pollicis brevis. To measure extension (hyperextension) the centre of the goniometer is placed over the posterior aspect of the joint, with the proximal arm in line with the metacarpal and the distal arm in line with the proximal phalanx.

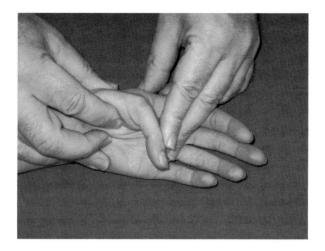

Fig 10.6 Determination of the range of flexion at the metacarpophalangeal joint of the thumb.

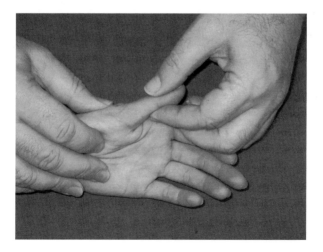

Fig 10.7 Determination of the range of extension at the metacarpophalangeal joint of the thumb.

Abduction

With the subject sitting, the forearm mid pronated/supinated with the medial border resting on a supporting surface, the wrist and carpometacarpal joints in neutral flexion/extension and abduction/adduction, the interphalangeal joint in neutral flexion/extension and the 1st metacarpal stabilised with the medial border of the hand resting on a supporting surface the metacarpophalangeal joint is abducted (Fig. 10.8). The final resistance to movement is firm due to tension in the medial joint capsule and collateral ligament. To measure abduction the centre of the goniometer is placed over the posterior aspect of the joint, with the proximal arm in line with the metacarpal and the distal arm in line with the proximal phalanx.

Opposition

With the subject sitting, the forearm supinated and resting on a supporting surface, the wrist in neutral flexion/extension and abduction/adduction, the interphalangeal joint of the thumb in neutral and the 5th metacarpal stabilised with the hand resting on a supporting surface the thumb is opposed (Fig. 10.9). The final resistance to movement may be soft, due to compression of the thenar eminence against the palm of the hand, or firm, due to tension in the joint capsule and extensor pollicis brevis. The distance between the tips of the thumb and little finger or the distance between the tip of the thumb and the base of the 5th metacarpal is measured using a ruler. If movement is allowed at the metacarpophalangeal and interphalangeal joints of the little finger the tips of the thumb and little finger usually meet.

The thumb can also be opposed to the index, middle and ring fingers.

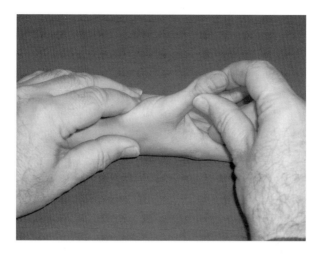

Fig 10.8 Determination of the range of abduction at the metacarpophalangeal joint of the thumb.

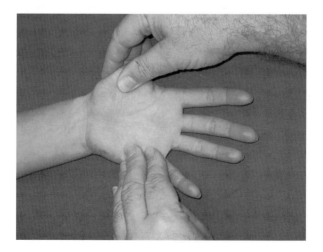

Fig 10.9 Determination of the range of opposition at the metacarpophalangeal joint of the thumb.

Interphalangeal joint
Anatomy

A hinge synovial joint between the pulley-shaped proximal phalanx and the reciprocally shaped base of the distal phalanx (Fig. 10.10). A loose fibrous capsule strengthened at the sides by the collateral ligaments and partly replaced anteriorly and posteriorly by the palmar ligament and extensor expansion of the tendon of extensor pollicis longus respectively, surrounds the joint.

Range of movement
Flexion and extension

Movement is about a transverse axis through the proximal phalanx nine-tenths of its length from the base (Youm *et al.*, 1978). The range of flexion is approximately 90°, while extension is usually no more than 10°; however, passive hyperextension may be marked in some individuals.

Accessory movement

An accessory anteroposterior gliding of the distal phalanx against the proximal may be elicited.

Evaluation of range of motion
Flexion

With the subject sitting, the forearm supinated and resting on a supporting surface, the wrist and carpometacarpal joints in neutral flexion/extension and abduction/adduction, the metacarpophalangeal joint in neutral flexion/extension and the proximal phalanx stabilised with the hand resting on a supporting surface the interphalangeal joint is flexed (Fig. 10.11). The final resistance to movement is usually firm due to tension in the collateral ligaments and posterior joint capsule, but may be hard due to contact between the palmar aspect of the distal phalanx, the palmar ligament and the proximal phalanx. To measure flexion the centre of the goniometer is placed over the posterior aspect of the joint, with the proximal arm in line with the proximal phalanx and the distal arm in line with the distal phalanx.

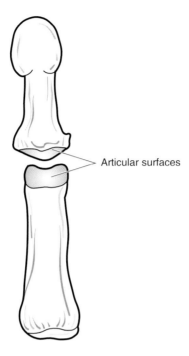

Articular surfaces

Fig 10.10   The articular surfaces of the interphalangeal joint of the thumb.

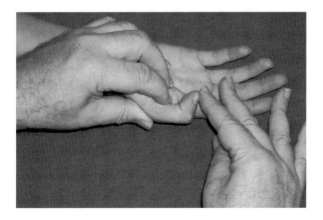

Fig 10.11   Determination of the range of flexion at the interphalangeal joint of the thumb.

Extension

With the subject sitting, the forearm supinated and resting on a supporting surface, the wrist and carpometacarpal joints in neutral flexion/extension and abduction/adduction, the metacarpophalangeal joint in neutral flexion/extension and the proximal phalanx stabilised with the hand resting on a supporting surface the interphalangeal joint is extended (Fig. 10.12). The final resistance to movement is usually firm due to tension in the anterior joint capsule and palmar ligament. To measure extension the centre of the goniometer is placed over the posterior aspect of the joint, with the proximal arm in line with the proximal phalanx and the distal arm in line with the distal phalanx.

FINGERS
Common carpometacarpal joint

An irregular line of plane synovial joints between the distal row of carpal bones and the bases of the 2nd to 5th metacarpals. The 2nd metacarpal articulates with the trapezium, trapezoid and capitate; the 3rd with the capitate; the 4th with the capitate and hamate; and the 5th with the hamate. The joint is surrounded by a fibrous capsule strengthened by dorsal and palmar carpometacarpal ligaments. It is extremely stable, providing a firm base between the joints of the wrist and those of the hand.

Little movement is possible at the joint, being flexion only: the 2nd and 3rd metacarpals are essentially immobile, the 4th glides slightly against the hamate, while only the 5th has any appreciable gliding movement against the hamate seen during a tight grasp and in opposition of the thumb to the little finger.

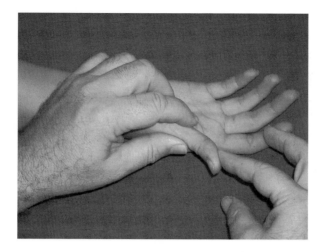

Fig 10.12 Determination of the range of extension at the interphalangeal joint of the thumb.

Metacarpophalangeal joints

Anatomy

Condyloid synovial joints between the rounded biconvex head of the metacarpal and the shallow oval concavity of the base of the proximal phalanx (Fig. 10.13). The metacarpal head is wider anteriorly than posteriorly and has a greater curvature transversely than anteroposteriorly. The base of the proximal phalanx has a smaller articular surface than the metacarpal, being increased by the fibrocartilaginous palmar ligament attached to its anterior surface.

Each joint is surrounded by a fibrous capsule strengthened on each side by collateral ligaments, replaced anteriorly and posteriorly by the palmar ligament and extensor expansion of the tendon of extensor digitorum respectively.

Range of movement

The shape of the joint surfaces permits active movement in two planes, flexion/extension in the sagittal plane and abduction/adduction in the frontal plane, as well as passive axial rotation: however, active rotation is possible in the little finger.

Flexion and extension

Occurs about a transverse axis through the head of the metacarpal nine-tenths of its length from the base (Youm *et al.*, 1978). The active range of flexion approaches 90° for the index finger increasing to 110° for the little finger: flexion of one joint in isolation is limited due to the tension developed in the deep transverse metacarpal ligaments. The active range of extension is 45° (AAOS, 1994), but is highly variable. The total active range of flexion and extension has been reported as being 148°, 145°, 149° and 152° for the index, middle, ring and little fingers; the passive ranges being 155°, 151°, 159° and 172° respectively (Youm *et al.*, 1978).

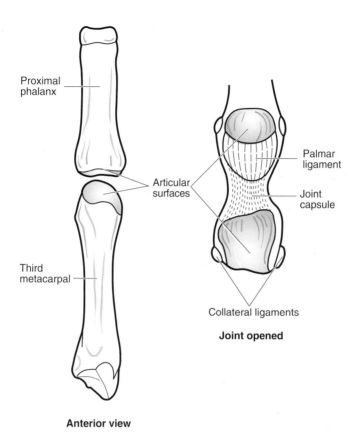

Proximal phalanx

Third metacarpal

Articular surfaces

Palmar ligament

Joint capsule

Collateral ligaments

Joint opened

Anterior view

Fig 10.13 The articular surfaces of the metacarpophalangeal joints of the fingers.

Abduction and adduction

Takes place about an anteroposterior axis through the head of the meta-carpal, the movement being away from (abduction) or towards (adduction) the middle finger: it is easier and has a greater range when the finger is extended (Youm *et al.*, 1978). The total active/passive range of abduction and adduction is 50°/62°, 40°/53°, 38°/55° and 57°/68° for the index, middle, ring and little fingers respectively (Youm *et al.*, 1978).

Evaluation of the range of motion

Flexion

With the subject sitting, the forearm in mid pronation/supination and rest-ing on a supporting surface, the wrist in neutral flexion/extension and abduction/adduction, the metacarpophalangeal joint in neutral abduc-tion/adduction and the metacarpal stabilised with the hand resting on a supporting surface the metacarpophalangeal joint is flexed (Fig. 10.14): the other metacarpophalangeal joints should be free to move so as not to restrict movement. The final resistance to movement is usually firm due to tension in the posterior joint capsule and collateral ligaments, but may be hard due to contact between the palmar aspect of the proximal phalanx and the metacarpal. To measure flexion the centre of the goniometer is placed over the posterior aspect of the metacarpophalangeal joint, with the proximal arm in line with the metacarpal and the distal arm in line with the proximal phalanx.

Extension

With the subject sitting, the forearm in mid pronation/supination and resting on a supporting surface, the wrist in neutral flexion/extension and abduction/adduction, the metacarpophalangeal joint in neutral abduction/adduction and the metacarpal stabilised with the hand resting on a sup-porting surface the metacarpophalangeal joint is extended (Fig. 10.15): the other metacarpophalangeal joints should be free to move so as not to restrict movement. The final resistance to movement is firm due to tension in the anterior joint capsule and palmar ligament. To measure extension the centre of the goniometer is placed over the posterior aspect of the metacarpophalangeal joint, with the proximal arm in line with the metacarpal and the distal arm in line with the proximal phalanx.

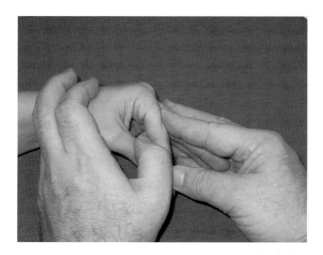

Fig 10.14 Determination of the range of flexion at the metacarpophalangeal joint of the index finger.

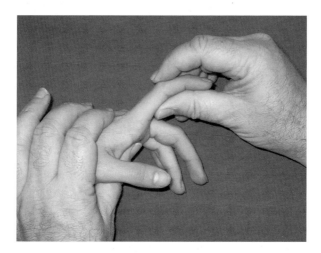

Fig 10.15 Determination of the range of extension at the metacarpophalangeal joint of the index finger.

Abduction

With the subject sitting, the forearm pronated and resting on a supporting surface, the wrist in neutral flexion/extension and abduction/adduction, the metacarpophalangeal joint in neutral flexion/extension and the metacarpal stabilised with the hand resting on a supporting surface the metacarpophalangeal joint is abducted (Fig. 10.16). The final resistance to movement is firm due to tension in the collateral ligaments, the fascia of the web space between the fingers and the appropriate palmar interosseous. To measure abduction the centre of the goniometer is placed flat over the posterior aspect of the metacarpophalangeal joint, with the proximal arm in line with the metacarpal and the distal arm in line with the proximal phalanx.

Adduction

With the subject sitting, the forearm pronated and resting on a supporting surface, the wrist in neutral flexion/extension and abduction/adduction, the metacarpophalangeal joint in neutral flexion/extension and the metacarpal stabilised with the hand resting on a supporting surface the metacarpophalangeal joint is adducted (Fig. 10.17). The final resistance to movement is firm due to tension in the collateral ligaments, the fascia of the web space between the fingers and the appropriate dorsal interosseous. To measure adduction the centre of the goniometer is placed flat over the posterior aspect of the metacarpophalangeal joint, with the proximal arm in line with the metacarpal and the distal arm in line with the proximal phalanx.

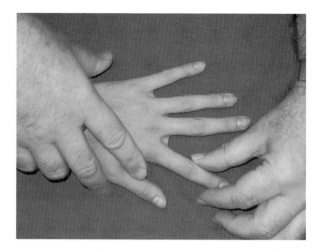

Fig 10.16 Determination of the range of abduction at the metacarpophalangeal joint of the index finger.

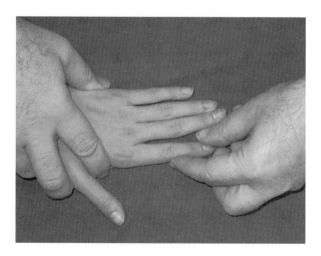

Fig 10.17 Determination of the range of adduction at the metacarpophalangeal joint of the index finger.

Interphalangeal joints
Anatomy

A hinge synovial joint between the pulley-shaped head of the proximal (middle) phalanx and the reciprocally shaped base of the middle (distal) phalanx (Fig. 10.18). A loose fibrous capsule strengthened at the sides by collateral ligaments and partly replaced anteriorly and posteriorly by the palmar ligament and extensor expansion of the tendon of extensor digitorum respectively, surrounds each joint.

Range of movement
Flexion and extension

Movement is about a transverse axis through the proximal (middle) phalanx nine-tenths of its length from the base (Youm et al., 1978). The axes assume increasing obliquity for the middle, ring and little fingers running from lateral and distal to medial and proximal, being approximately perpendicular to the groove on the phalangeal head. The range of flexion is greater than 90° for all proximal interphalangeal joints increasing towards the little finger, which can flex 135°. At the distal interphalangeal joint the range of flexion is 90° for the little finger gradually decreasing to the index finger. Extension at the interphalangeal joints is limited, being approximately 10° at the distal and 5° at the proximal joints.

Accessory movement

Accessory anteroposterior gliding can be elicited at each joint of all four fingers.

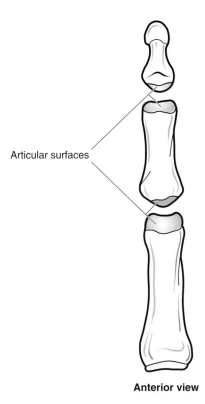

Articular surfaces

Anterior view

Fig 10.18 The articular surfaces of the interphalangeal joints of the fingers.

Evaluation of range of motion
Proximal interphalangeal joint
Flexion

With the subject sitting, the forearm mid pronated/supinated and resting on a supporting surface, the wrist and metacarpophalangeal joints in neutral flexion/extension and abduction/adduction and the proximal phalanx stabilised with the hand resting on a supporting surface the proximal interphalangeal joint is flexed (Fig. 10.19). The final resistance to movement is usually hard due to contact between the palmar aspects of the middle and proximal phalanges; however it may be firm, due to tension in the posterior joint capsule and collateral ligaments, or soft, due to compression of the soft tissue between the middle and proximal phalanges. To measure flexion the centre of the goniometer is placed over the posterior aspect of the proximal interphalangeal joint, with the proximal and distal arms in line with the proximal and middle phalanges respectively.

Extension

With the subject sitting, the forearm mid pronated/supinated and resting on a supporting surface, the wrist and metacarpophalangeal joints in neutral flexion/extension and abduction/adduction and the proximal phalanx stabilised with the hand resting on a supporting surface the proximal interphalangeal joint is extended (Fig. 10.20). The final resistance to movement is firm due to tension in the anterior joint capsule and palmar ligament. To measure extension the centre of the goniometer is placed over the posterior aspect of the proximal interphalangeal joint, with the proximal and distal arms in line with the proximal and middle phalanges respectively.

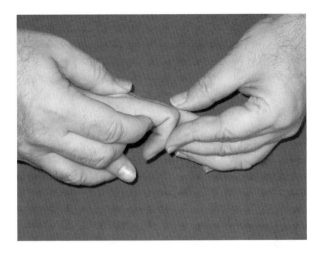

Fig 10.19 Determination of the range of flexion at the proximal interphalangeal joint of the index finger.

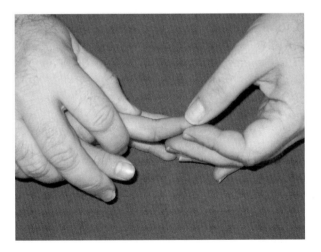

Fig 10.20 Determination of the range of extension at the proximal interphalangeal joint of the index finger.

Distal interphalangeal joint

Flexion

With the subject sitting, the forearm mid pronated/supinated and resting on a supporting surface, the wrist and metacarpophalangeal joints in neutral flexion/extension and abduction/adduction, the proximal interphalangeal joint flexed to 90° and the middle phalanx stabilised with the hand resting on a supporting surface the distal interphalangeal joint is abducted (Fig. 10.21). The final resistance to movement is firm due to tension in the posterior joint capsule and collateral ligaments. To measure flexion the centre of the goniometer is placed over the posterior aspect of the distal interphalangeal joint, with the proximal and distal arms in line with the middle and distal phalanges respectively.

Extension

With the subject sitting, the forearm mid pronated/supinated and resting on a supporting surface, the wrist and metacarpophalangeal joints in neutral flexion/extension and abduction/adduction, the proximal interphalangeal joint flexed to 90° and the middle phalanx stabilised with the hand resting on a supporting surface the distal interphalangeal joint is extended (Fig. 10.22). The final resistance to movement is firm due to tension in the anterior joint capsule and palmar ligament. To measure extension the centre of the goniometer is placed over the posterior aspect of the distal interphalangeal joint, with the proximal and distal arms in line with the middle and distal phalanges respectively.

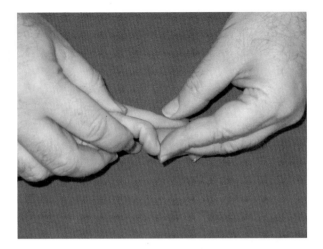

Fig 10.21 Determination of the range of flexion at the distal interphalangeal joint of the index finger.

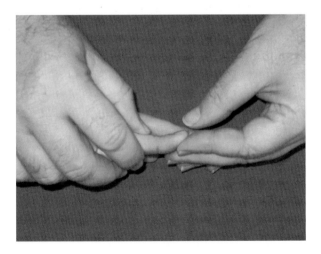

Fig 10.22 Determination of the range of extension at the distal interphalangeal joint of the index finger.

11 Pelvic girdle

The pelvic girdle provides articulation of the lower limbs with the trunk (Fig. 11.1). It consists of a ring of bone comprising the two innominates and the sacrum: the innominates articulate with each other anteriorly at the symphysis pubis (a secondary cartilaginous joint) and with the sacrum at the synovial sacroiliac joint on each side. The articulation with the lower limbs is via the acetabulum of the hip joint (Chapter 12) and with the vertebral column via the lumbosacral joint (Chapter 16).

SACROILIAC JOINT
Anatomy

The joint is formed between the L-shaped irregular auricular surfaces of the sacrum and ilium: the surfaces are broader superiorly than inferiorly

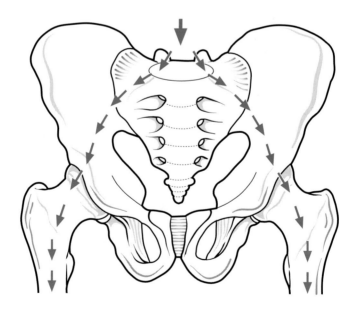

Fig 11.1 The articulation of the pelvic girdle with the vertebral column and lower limbs, also showing the transfer of weight from the vertebral column through the pelvis to the femur.

(Fig. 11.2). The sacral surface is covered with hyaline cartilage, while that on the ilium is covered with fibrocartilage. With increasing age, especially in males, the joint cavity becomes partially, or occasionally completely, obliterated by fibrocartilaginous adhesions: in the elderly there may be bony fusion.

A fibrous capsule surrounds the joint being reinforced by strong anterior and posterior sacroiliac ligaments: accessory ligaments (sacrotuberous, sacrospinous) provide additional stability.

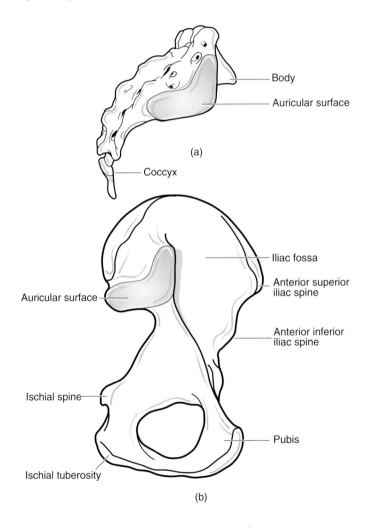

Fig 11.2 The articular surfaces of the sacroiliac joint (a) on the sacrum, (b) on the innominate.

Movement

The irregular nature of the joint surfaces, together with the strong associated ligaments, permit little movement. Nevertheless, both gliding and rotatory movements are possible so that when standing compared with lying supine the sacrum moves downwards some 2 mm and undergoes 5° of forward rotation. Sudden forward flexion can tear the posterior sacroiliac ligaments with the possibility of joint dislocation.

During the latter stages of pregnancy the ligaments of the joint become more lax permitting greater movement: childbirth sees a complex pattern of movement, similar to nodding of the head, which serves to increase the diameters of the pelvic inlet and outlet. Initially the sacral promontory moves posterosuperiorly, increasing the anteroposterior diameter of the pelvic inlet by 3–13 mm (Fig. 11.3a). After the foetal head has entered the pelvic canal the sacral promontory moves anteroinferiorly, increasing the anteroposterior diameter of the pelvic canal by 15–18 mm (Fig. 11.3b).

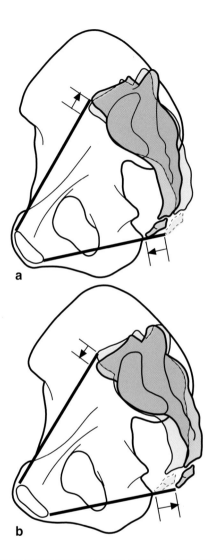

Fig 11.3 Movement of the sacrum against the innominate: (a) to increase the diameter of the pelvic inlet; (b) to increase the diameter of the pelvic outlet.

Accessory movements can be demonstrated with the subject lying prone and placing the heel of the hand over the apex of the sacrum. With downward pressure a small degree of rotation is possible (Fig. 11.4).

SYMPHYSIS PUBIS
Anatomy

A secondary cartilaginous joint between the medial surfaces of the pubic bones of each innominate (Fig. 11.5). The articular surfaces are covered with a thin layer of hyaline cartilage joined by an interpubic fibrocartilaginous disc, thicker in females than males. A fluid-filled cavity appears posterosuperiorly early in life, which enlarges to extend throughout the disc in females.

The joint is reinforced by fibrous thickenings superiorly (superior pubic ligament), inferiorly (arcuate pubic ligament) and anteriorly (anterior pubic ligament) by the decussating tendinous fibres of rectus femoris, external oblique and adductor longus anteriorly.

Movement

No movement is normally possible at the joint; however, during pregnancy ligament laxity may permit up to 2 mm separation of the symphysis pubis. Absorption of the bone adjacent to the joint may also facilitate separation.

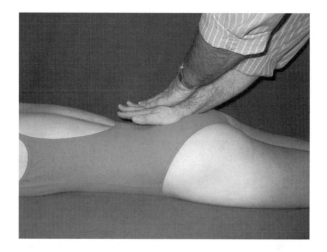

Fig 11.4 With the subject lying prone accessory rotatory movements at the sacroiliac joint can be elicited by applying pressure with the heel of the hand over the apex of the sacrum.

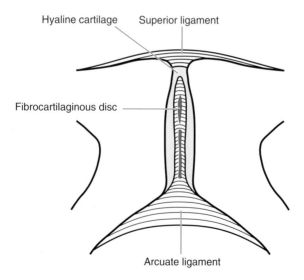

Hyaline cartilage   Superior ligament

Fibrocartilaginous disc

Arcuate ligament

Fig 11.5 The articular surfaces of the symphysis pubis.

LUMBOSACRAL JOINT
Anatomy

The articulation is between L5 and S1 (Fig. 11.6): the bodies by a secondary cartilaginous joint and the articular facets by synovial joints. An intervertebral disc is situated between the bodies, with anterior and posterior longitudinal ligaments also connecting the bodies: ligamenta flava, interspinous and supraspinous ligaments connect the neural arches. Further details of vertebral articulations are given on page 168.

The lumbosacral joint is further reinforced by iliolumbar and lateral lumbosacral ligaments.

Range of movements

Flexion, extension and lateral flexion are all possible at the joint. In the young a small degree of axial rotation may also be possible; however, this soon becomes minimal.

Flexion and extension

Between ages 2 and 13 the lumbosacral joint may be responsible for as much as 75% of the total movement of the lumbar spine, with the average range of movement being 18°: this is greatly reduced after age 35.

Lateral flexion

Lateral flexion decreases from approximately 7° in the child to 1° in adults and 0° in the elderly.

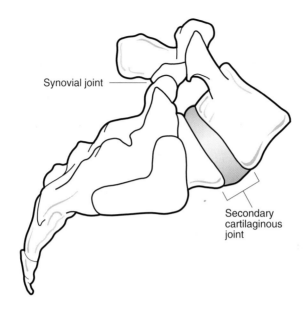

Synovial joint

Secondary
cartilaginous
joint

Fig 11.6   Anatomy of the lumbosacral articulation.

12 Hip joint

ANATOMY

The hip joint is a synovial ball-and-socket joint between the head of the femur and the acetabulum of the pelvis. It is a major weight-bearing joint connecting the lower limb to the trunk, supporting and transferring body weight from the trunk to the lower limb during locomotor activities, as well as permitting a wide range of movements.

During development the relationship between the head and neck of the femur and the shaft changes in both the frontal and horizontal planes. At birth the head and neck are abducted some 150° (angle of inclination) and laterally rotated 25° (angle of anteversion) with respect to the shaft. With increasing age these angles decrease to average adult values of 125° inclination and 10° anteversion (Fig. 12.1a). These changes have important implications for joint stability during the growth: there are also considerable individual and racial variations in these angles.

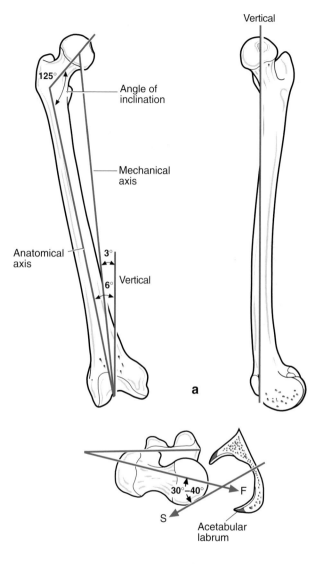

Fig 12.1 The relation between the head and neck of the femur in the adult: (a) viewed from the front and medially; (b) viewed from above showing the relationship with the acetabulum of the pelvis.

The head of the femur is ellipsoid, being slightly compressed anteroposteriorly, forming approximately two-thirds of a sphere: posteromedially the fovea capitis is non-articular (Fig. 12.2). The acetabulum is an hemispherical depression on the outer surface of the pelvis, which faces laterally, anteriorly and inferiorly, surrounded and deepened by the acetabular labrum: the deep central area is non-articular (Fig. 12.2). Although reciprocally curved the two articular surfaces are not congruent at low loads, but become more so with increasing loads. Due to the orientation of the acetabulum and the anteversion of the femoral neck the two articular surfaces are not coincident (Fig. 12.1b): the anterior and anterosuperior aspects of the femoral head articulate with the joint capsule.

The joint capsule is extremely strong, attaching proximally to the margin of the acetabulum and transverse ligament, which bridges the acetabular notch, and distally to the intertrochanteric line and midway along the neck of the femur posteriorly. The iliofemoral and pubofemoral ligaments reinforce the capsule anteriorly, while the ischiofemoral ligament does so posteriorly; the deep fibres of rectus femoris and gluteus minimus strengthen the capsule anteromedially and laterally respectively.

Stability of the joint is determined by the shape of the articular surfaces and acetabular labrum, the strength of the joint capsule and its associated ligaments, as well as muscles crossing the joint, especially those running transversely.

RANGES OF MOVEMENT

Movement is possible in all three planes: flexion–extension in the sagittal plane about a mediolateral axis, abduction–adduction in the coronal plane about an anteroposterior axis, and medial and lateral rotation in the transverse plane about a vertical axis. The three axes intersect at the centre of the femoral head. The vertical (mechanical) axis of the femur is represented by a line joining the centre of the femoral head to the centre of the knee joint (Fig. 12.1a). Because the femoral neck and head is angled against the shaft all movements at the hip joint involve conjoint rotation of the femoral head.

Flexion and extension

The total range of active flexion and extension is approximately 135° (Roach and Miles, 1991), with flexion being freer (120°) than extension (15°). Passive movement can increase the range to 145° of flexion and 30° extension: extension beyond 30° is not normally possible as the capsular ligaments become increasingly taut, pulling the femoral head tightly against the acetabulum. The range of both flexion and extension change

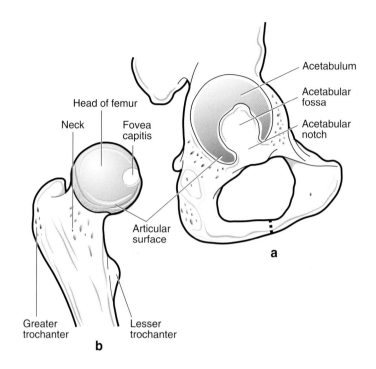

Fig 12.2 The articular surfaces of (a) the head of the femur and (b) the acetabulum.

Table 12.1 Required range of movement at the hip during various activities (adapted from Livingston *et al.*, 1991)

Activity	Max range required
Walking on level surfaces	30° flexion
	10° extension
	5° abduction
	5° adduction
	5° medial rotation
	5° lateral rotation
Ascending stairs	65° flexion
	5° extension
Descending stairs	65° flexion
	5° extension
Sitting	90° flexion (minimum)
Tying shoe laces	50° flexion

with age. In neonates flexion is 138° (Watanabe *et al.*, 1979); however, all newborns and young infants are unable to extend the hip to the neutral position from full flexion: this limitation is some 30° (Forero *et al.*, 1989), but may be as much as 46° at birth (Waugh *et al.*, 1983). By 4 or 5 years of age active extension of 30° is possible (Svenningsen *et al.*, 1989). With increasing age the range of flexion and extension gradually decreases to adult values, but thereafter remains relatively constant until age 70 after which a decrease in both active and passive range of motion has been observed (James and Parker, 1989).

Abduction and adduction

Abduction and adduction are free in all positions of the lower limb with a total range of 75°: 45° abduction and 30° adduction. Abduction is greatest with the hip partly flexed, being limited by tension in the adductors and medial part of the iliofemoral and pubofemoral ligaments, while adduction is easier with the hip flexed than extended, being limited by the opposite limb, the abductors and lateral part of the iliofemoral ligament. In young children abduction may approach 60° (Phelps *et al.*, 1985), decreasing to adult values from age 6, while adduction, except in the newborn when it is only some 6° (Drews *et al.*, 1984), remains relatively constant at 30°.

Medial and lateral rotation

Rotation at the hip takes place about the mechanical axis of the femur, consequently in medial rotation the femoral shaft moves anteriorly and medially while in lateral rotation it moves posteriorly and laterally. Rotation is freer when the hip is flexed than extended, with lateral rotation being more powerful than medial rotation. The total range of rotation in adults is 90°, 45° medially and 45° laterally; however, with increasing age the range decreases to 60° (Roach and Miles, 1991), the decrease being equal in both directions. In neonates, infants and young children the total range of rotation is much greater than in adults with lateral rotation initially being the greater but from age 4 medial rotation is greater than that laterally. In neonates rotation is 92° laterally and 76° medially (Forero *et al.*, 1989), decreasing to 46° and 55° respectively by age 4 (Svenningsen *et al.*, 1989) and 43° and 48° at age 11 (Svenningsen *et al.*, 1989).

Females have been observed to be more mobile for most movements of the hip than males at all ages (Allander *et al.*, 1974; James and Parker, 1989). The ranges of motion associated with some common activities are given in Table 12.1.

EVALUATION OF RANGE OF MOTION
Flexion

With the subject lying supine, the hip in neutral abduction/adduction and rotation and the knee extended, the hip is flexed while the pelvis is stabilised (Fig. 12.3): the opposite hip is flexed sufficiently to flatten the lumbar spine. As flexion approaches its maximum the knee is allowed to flex to prevent tension in the hamstrings limiting the movement. Maximum active flexion is reached when the pelvis begins to rotate; maximum passive flexion occurs when the anterior thigh makes contact with the lower abdominal wall. The final resistance to movement is usually soft because of the soft tissue contact; however, it may be firm due to tension in the posterior joint capsule and gluteus maximus. To measure hip flexion the centre of the goniometer is placed over the lateral aspect of the greater trochanter, with the proximal arm aligned over the lateral midline of the pelvis and the distal arm in line with the lateral epicondyle of the femur.

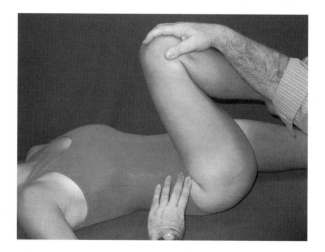

Fig 12.3 Determination of the range of flexion at the hip joint with subject lying supine.

Extension

The subject lies prone with the hip in neutral abduction/adduction and rotation and the knee extended, the hip is then extended (Fig. 12.4). Maximum extension is taken as when the pelvis begins to rotate. The final resistance to movement is firm because of tension developed in the anterior joint capsule and the iliofemoral, pubofemoral and ischiofemoral ligaments: there may also be tension in muscles that flex the hip. To measure hip extension, the centre of the goniometer is placed over the lateral aspect of the greater trochanter, with the proximal arm aligned over the lateral midline of the pelvis and the distal arm in line with the lateral epicondyle of the femur.

Alternatively the subject supports the trunk on the examination table with the opposite hip flexed and the foot on the ground (Fig. 12.5). Movement of the pelvis is more easily determined; however, this method is awkward in adults although easier to perform in children.

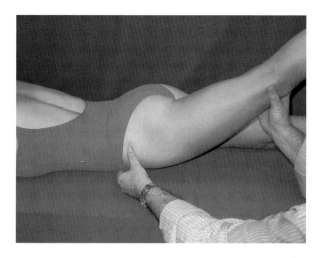

Fig 12.4 Determination of the range of extension at the hip joint with the subject lying prone.

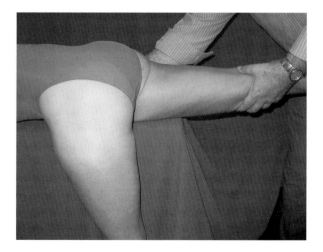

Fig 12.5 Determination of the range of extension at the hip joint with the subject's opposite hip flexed and foot on the ground.

Abduction

With the subject supine, the hip in neutral flexion/extension and rotation and the knee extended, the hip is abducted (Fig. 12.6): the pelvis is stabilised to prevent rotation and lateral tilting. During the movement the ankle is held to prevent lateral rotation of the hip. Maximum abduction is reached when the pelvis starts to tilt, determined by placing the hand over the opposite anterior superior iliac spine (ASIS), or when there is lateral flexion of the spine. The final resistance to movement is firm because of tension in the joint capsule, pubofemoral and medial band of the iliofemoral ligaments, as well as in the adductor muscles. To measure abduction the centre of the goniometer is placed over the anterior superior iliac spine, with the proximal arm aligned with the opposite ASIS and the distal arm in line with the midline of the patella.

Abduction can also be measured with the hip flexed at 90° (Fig. 12.7); however, care must be taken to abduct the flexed hip and not laterally rotate it. Measuring abduction in flexion is useful in neonates and young infants.

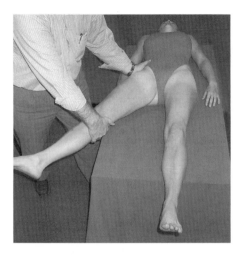

Fig 12.6 Determination of the range of abduction of the hip joint with the subject lying supine.

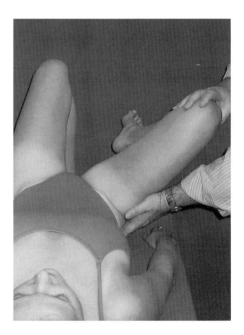

Fig 12.7 Determination of the range of abduction at the hip joint with the subject lying supine and the hip flexed to 90°.

Adduction

With the subject supine, the hip in neutral flexion/extension and rotation and the knee extended, the hip is adducted (Fig. 12.8): the pelvis is stabilised to prevent rotation and lateral tilting. During the movement the ankle is held to prevent lateral rotation of the hip. Maximum adduction is reached when the pelvis starts to tilt, determined by placing the hand over the opposite ASIS, or when there is lateral flexion of the spine. The final resistance to movement is firm because of tension in the joint capsule, ischiofemoral and lateral band of the iliofemoral ligaments, as well as in the abductor muscles. To measure adduction the centre of the goniometer is placed over the anterior superior iliac spine, with the proximal arm aligned with the opposite ASIS and the distal arm in line with the midline of the patella.

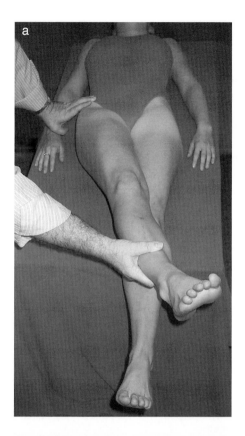

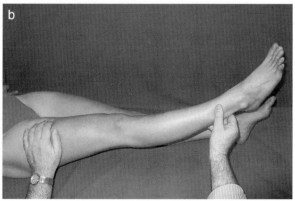

Fig 12.8 Determination of the range of adduction at the hip joint with the subject lying supine: (a) viewed from above; (b) viewed from the side.

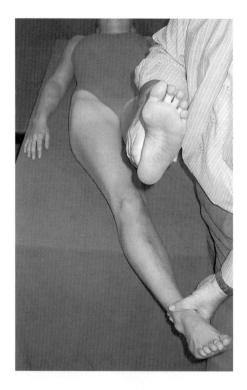

Fig 12.9 Determination of the range of adduction at the hip joint with the subject lying supine with the opposite hip flexed and the limb supported.

Alternatively, the opposite limb can be flexed and supported (Fig. 12.9). The final resistance to movement is firm because of tension in the joint capsule and lateral band of the iliofemoral ligament, as well as the muscles which abduct the hip.

Medial rotation

With the subject sitting with the legs hanging freely over the side of the supporting surface, the hip in neutral abduction/adduction and 90° flexion, the hip is medially rotated by moving the leg away from the midline (Fig. 12.10). The distal end of the femur is stabilised to prevent adduction and further flexion at the hip: a rolled towel placed under the distal femur helps maintain the femur horizontal. During movement rotation and lateral tilting of the pelvis must also be prevented. Maximum medial rotation is reached when the pelvis begins to lift off the supporting surface. The final resistance to movement is firm because of tension in the joint capsule and ischiofemoral ligament, as well as the lateral rotators. The centre of the goniometer is placed over the front of the patella, with one arm aligned perpendicular to the floor or supporting surface and the other arm in line with the tibial tuberosity and midway between the two malleoli.

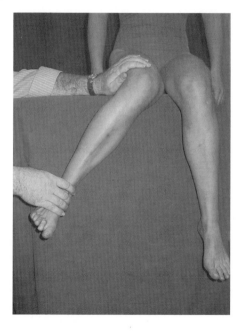

Fig 12.10 Determination of the range of medial rotation at the hip joint with the subject seated.

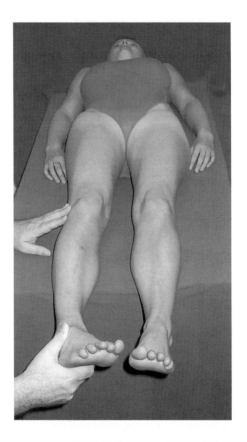

Fig 12.11 Determination of the range of medial rotation at the hip joint with the subject lying supine.

Medial rotation may also be measured with the subject lying supine or prone. With the subject lying supine, the hip in neutral flexion/extension and abduction/adduction, the knee extended and ankle in neutral plantarflexion/dorsiflexion, medial rotation is measured by rotating the foot towards the midline (Fig. 12.11). The centre of the goniometer is placed over the centre of the heel, with one arm perpendicular to the supporting surface and the other in line with the second toe. With the subject prone,

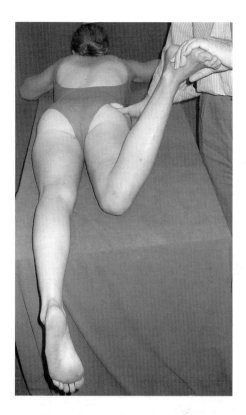

Fig 12.12 Determination of the range of medial rotation at the hip joint with the subject lying prone and the knee flexed to 90°.

the hip in neutral flexion/extension and abduction/adduction and the knee flexed 90°, medial rotation is measured by rotating the leg away from the midline (Fig. 12.12). The centre of the goniometer is placed over the front of the patella, with the one arm aligned perpendicular to the supporting surface and the other arm in line with the tibial tuberosity and midway between the two malleoli.

Lateral rotation

The testing positions and goniometer placements are similar to those outlined for medial rotation. With the subject sitting with the legs hanging freely over the side of the supporting surface, the hip is laterally rotated by rotating the leg towards the midline (Fig. 12.13). Maximum lateral rotation is reached when the pelvis begins to lift off the supporting surface. The final resistance to movement is firm because of tension in the joint capsule and iliofemoral and pubofemoral ligaments, as well as in muscles which produce medial rotation.

With the subject supine lateral rotation is measured by rotating the foot away from the midline (Fig. 12.14), while with the subject prone it is determined by rotating the leg towards the midline (Fig. 12.15).

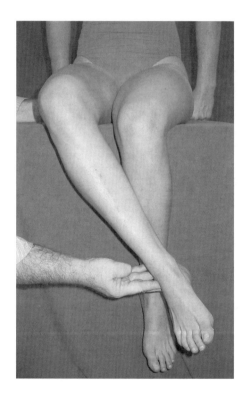

Fig 12.13 Determination of the range of lateral rotation at the hip joint with the subject seated.

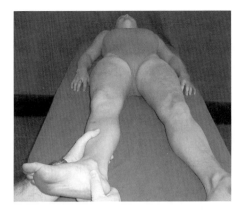

Fig 12.14 Determination of the range of lateral rotation at the hip joint with the subject lying supine.

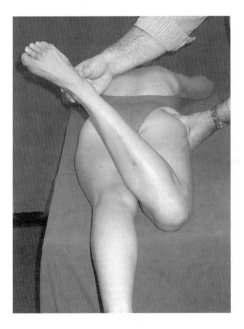

Fig 12.15 Determination of the range of lateral rotation at the hip joint with the subject lying prone and the knee flexed to 90°.

13 Knee joint

ANATOMY

The knee joint is a major weight-bearing joint of the lower limb, and as such is the largest and one of the most complex joints in the body. It is a synovial bicondylar modified hinge joint consisting of two distinct articulations, the tibiofemoral and patellofemoral joints. The joint axis is horizontal, being in the frontal plane.

The tibiofemoral articulation is between the relatively flat tibial condyles and the biconvex femoral condyles (Fig. 13.1). The tibial condyles are shallow concavities, with the medial being the larger, separated by the intercondylar eminence: the tibial surface as a whole has a slight posteroinferior inclination with respect to the horizontal. The two femoral condyles are separated from each other by the intercondylar notch posteriorly and the patellar surface anteriorly. The long axes of the two condyles diverge posteriorly, with the lateral being the longer.

The patellofemoral articulation is between the posterior surface of the patella and the patella surface of the femur (Fig. 13.1). On the patella a vertical ridge separates the larger lateral from the smaller medial articular surface. The patellar surface of the femur has a corresponding well-marked groove with a smaller medial and larger more prominent lateral articular surface.

The true joint capsule is large and loose, being reinforced by expansions from the surrounding muscles and their tendons to form a thick ligamentous sheath. The quadriceps tendon, its expansions and the patellar ligament reinforce the capsule anteriorly, the oblique and arcuate popliteal ligaments posteriorly, and the medial collateral ligament medially.

Anteroposterior stability of the joint is predominantly provided by the anterior and posterior cruciate ligaments (ACL, PCL), while the lateral collateral ligament and iliotibial tract, and sartorius, gracilis and semitendinosus essentially provide lateral and medial joint stability respectively. In addition to their role in providing anteroposterior stability the cruciate ligaments also provide some resistance to lateral (PCL) and medial (ACL) displacement.

The form of the two collateral ligaments of the knee joint differ greatly. The lateral collateral ligament is an independent rounded cord, while the

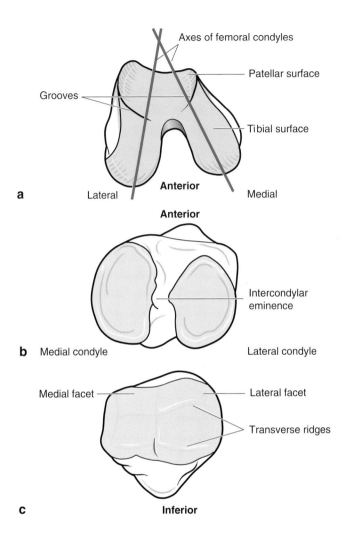

Axes of femoral condyles

Patellar surface

Grooves

Tibial surface

a   Lateral   **Anterior**   Medial

Anterior

Intercondylar eminence

b   Medial condyle   Lateral condyle

Medial facet   Lateral facet

Transverse ridges

c   **Inferior**

Fig 13.1   The articular surfaces of the knee joint: (a) the femur; (b) the tibia; (c) the patella.

medial collateral ligament is a strong flat band which blends with the joint capsule and whose deep fibres attach to the medial meniscus. The intra-capsular but extrasynovial cruciate ligaments consist of composite bands of fibres passing from tibia to femur, spiraling and twisting as they do so.

RANGES OF MOVEMENT

Due to the nature of its articulations the knee joint provides considerable stability, particularly in extension, yet it is also reasonably mobile, especially in flexion. At the tibiofemoral articulation motion takes place in all three planes, but the range of movement is greatest in the sagittal plane, i.e. flexion and extension.

Flexion and extension

The total range of active movement from full flexion to full extension is approximately 140° with the hip flexed (Boone and Azen, 1979; Roaas and Andersson, 1982) and 120° with the hip extended: the difference being due to the hamstrings losing some of their efficiency with hip extension (Kapandji, 1970). Passive movement at the joint can increase the total range to 160° allowing the heel to touch the buttock. According to Roach and Miles (1991) beyond the age of 40 active knee flexion decreases to 130°; however, they conclude that a loss of motion of more than 10% of the total range should be considered to be abnormal.

The initial 10–15° of flexion from the neutral position essentially involves rolling of the femoral condyles over the tibial condyles, beyond which the femoral condyles slide past a limited area on the tibial condyles. The rolling of the lateral femoral condyle may last until 20° of flexion.

Newborn children have been found to lack approximately 15 to 20° of knee extension (Waugh *et al.*, 1983; Drews *et al.*, 1984); however, by age 2 full extension is possible (Watanabe *et al.*, 1979) and by age 10 there is some 7° of hyperextension (Cheng *et al.*, 1991). During the remainder of childhood and throughout most of adulthood hyperextension, if present, is usually only of the order of a few degrees. (Hyperextension is extension beyond the extended straight leg position, i.e. the neutral joint position.)

During the last 10–15° of active extension an automatic rotation of the knee occurs whereby if the foot is fixed the femur medially rotates on the tibia: alternatively if the foot is free the tibia laterally rotates against the femur. Consequently, to enable flexion to begin the knee must undergo some degree of rotation opposite in direction to that which occurred in extension. This rotation accompanying full extension or the initial phase of flexion is not under voluntary control; it is entirely automatic.

The Helfet test can be used to determine whether lateral rotation of the tibia occurs during knee extension (Helfet, 1974); i.e. that the screw-home mechanism is intact. The test is performed with the subject sitting with the hip and knee flexed 90° and the leg hanging freely over the side of a supporting surface. The medial and lateral borders of the patella are marked on the skin, and lines drawn on the middle of the patella and the tibial tuberosity (Fig. 13.2), and the alignment of the tuberosity with the patella

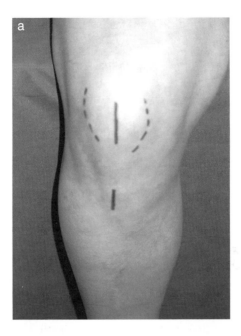

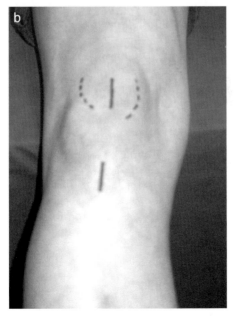

Fig 13.2 The Helfet test: (a) knee flexed; (b) knee extended.

checked. The knee is then extended and movement of the tibial tuberosity is observed. In a normal knee the tibial tuberosity moves laterally during extension and becomes aligned with the lateral half of the patella in full extension.

Medial and lateral rotation

Medial and lateral rotation occurs in the transverse plane and is influenced by the degree of flexion of the joint. With the knee fully extended little or no rotation is possible because of the interlocking of the tibial and femoral condyles. As the knee flexes rotation becomes possible, with the range increasing with increasing flexion and becoming maximum at 90° of flexion. Maximal active medial and lateral rotation is 30° and 45° respectively; these values can be increased to 35° and 50° if the movement is performed passively. Beyond 90° of knee flexion the total range of rotation decreases due to restrictions imposed by the soft tissues.

Abduction and adduction

Abduction and adduction motion in the frontal plane, although limited, is again influenced by the degree of knee joint flexion. In full extension no motion is possible, but passive abduction and adduction both increase up to 30° of knee flexion. Beyond 30° frontal plane motion again decreases due to soft tissue limitations.

The ranges of knee joint flexion associated with some common activities are given in Table 13.1, from which it can be seen that a range of at least 105° appears to be required in order to be able to carry out everyday activities. No difference has been reported in the range of knee joint motion between men and women.

Table 13.1 Knee flexion range of movement required in various activities (adapted from Laubenthal *et al.*, 1972; Livingston *et al.*, 1991; Jevsevar *et al.*, 1993)

Activity	Max range of flexion required (°)
Walking	65
slow (stance phase)	5
free (stance phase)	15
fast (stance phase)	20
Running (stance phase)	30
Ascending stairs	105
Descending stairs	105
Getting out of a chair	90
Sitting down	95
Tying shoe laces	105

Accessory movements are possible at the knee, their extent being determined by joint position and tension in the associated ligaments. In full extension no accessory movements are possible, however at 25° flexion a number of accessory movements can be demonstrated. The tibia can be moved anteriorly and posteriorly be pulling/pushing in the appropriate direction. In addition rotation of the tibia on the femur is possible beyond the available range by applying a firm rotatory force to the tibia: the tibia can also be rocked medially and laterally. It is also possible to pull the tibia away from the femur by applying a longitudinal force.

EVALUATION OF RANGE OF MOTION
Flexion

With the subject lying supine, the knee extended and the hip in neutral, the knee can be flexed: when the knee flexes the hip also flexes (Fig. 13.3). The final resistance to movement is usually soft because of contact of the soft tissues of the calf or heel and the thigh. The final resistance may, however, be firm due to tension developed in the vastus muscles. At approximately 90° of hip flexion the femur is stabilised to prevent further hip flexion. To measure the degree of flexion the centre of the goniometer is placed over the lateral epicondyle of the femur, with the proximal arm pointing towards the greater trochanter and the distal arm pointing towards the lateral malleolus.

Alternatively the subject can lie prone with the foot hanging over the end of the supporting surface so that the hip is in neutral (Fig. 13.4). The final resistance to movement, if not soft, is firm due to the tension developed in rectus femoris. The goniometer is aligned as for the supine position. In both positions care should be taken to stabilise the femur to prevent unwanted movements.

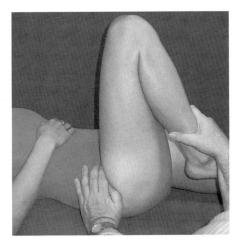

Fig 13.3 Determination of the range of flexion at the knee joint with the subject lying supine.

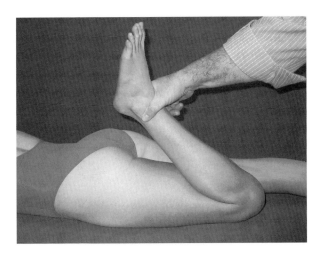

Fig 13.4 Determination of the range of flexion at the knee joint with the subject lying prone.

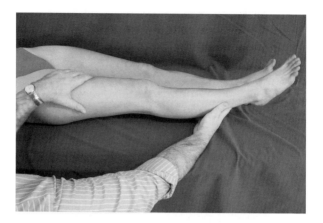

Fig 13.5 Determination of the range of extension at the knee joint with the subject lying supine.

Extension

The initial testing positions and goniometer alignment are the same as when measuring flexion (Fig. 13.5). The final resistance to movement is firm due to the tension in the posterior joint capsule, the oblique and arcuate popliteal ligaments, the collateral and cruciate ligaments.

Rotation

With the subject sitting with the leg hanging freely over the side of the supporting surface, the sole of the foot is held horizontally and the foot moved so that the toes point medially (medial rotation) (Fig. 13.6a) or laterally (lateral rotation) (Fig. 13.6b). The final resistance to rotatory movements is firm due to tension developed in the collateral ligaments (lateral rotation of the tibia), and cruciate ligaments (medial rotation of the tibia). The goniometer is placed with its centre over the centre of the heel with one arm in line with the long axis of the thigh and the other in line with the long axis of the foot.

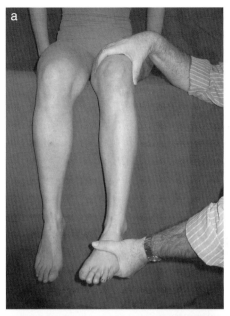

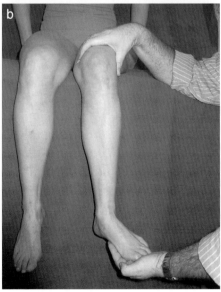

Fig 13.6 Determination of the range of rotation at the knee joint with the subject seated: (a) medial rotation; (b) lateral rotation.

Alternatively the subject can lie prone with the knee flexed to 90°. With the foot held horizontally it is moved so that the toes point medially (medial rotation) (Fig. 13.7a) or laterally (lateral rotation) (Fig. 13.7b). The goniometer is used as before.

Abduction/adduction

It is not possible to measure these movements in a normal joint.

JOINT LAXITY

Given the importance of the cruciate ligaments in providing anteroposterior stability at the knee joint, injury to these ligaments would be expected to have a major influence on joint laxity. Indeed injury to the ACL can have a profound effect on the stability, whereas injury to the PCL may have a minimal effect due to the action of the hamstring muscles. It is extremely important to have an accurate assessment of laxity so that appropriate recommendations can be made for treatment. Beighton *et al.* (1973) has observed that women have a greater degree of joint laxity than men at all ages; this should therefore be borne in mind when evaluating a joint laxity following potential injury.

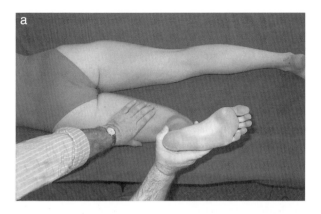

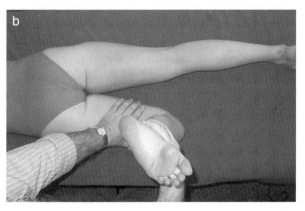

Fig 13.7 Determination of the range of rotation at the knee joint with the subject lying prone and the knee flexed to 90°: (a) medial rotation; (b) lateral rotation.

The classic sign of a ruptured ACL is an anterior draw sign with excessive mobility of the tibia on the femur at 90° of flexion. A normal knee would be expected to show 2–3 mm of movement; a knee joint with a completely ruptured ACL might exhibit up to 25 mm of movement. Unfortunately the anterior draw test often shows very little abnormal movement. However, if the test is performed with the knee at 10° of flexion then an abnormal movement in the anterior direction is seen with ACL damage: this examination is known as the Lachman test. There are several factors that can influence the Lachman test including: knee flexion angle, joint rotation, muscle tone, displacement force, and soft tissue restraints. Medial rotation of the tibia tightens the PCL thereby limiting the anterior draw effect; conversely lateral tibial rotation increases anterior displacement.

A new method of evaluating ACL stability has been reported by Adler *et al.* (1995), and is known as the Drop Leg Lachman test. The subject lies supine with the leg to be tested abducted so that the calf lies over the side of the supporting surface (Fig. 13.8); the knee is flexed to 25°. The angle of flexion and rotation of the leg are maintained by the examiner who holds the foot between their legs, while the patient's thigh is kept steady on the table using one hand: the leg is then extended and abducted, relaxing the hamstrings and tensor fascia lata. The examiner's free hand is then placed behind the subject's leg and an anterior force applied, as in the Lachman test. The test must be conducted with the subject relaxed, under anaesthesia if necessary.

The Drop Leg Lachman test has several advantages over the Lachman test in that it is easier to perform, is highly reproducible, allows bulky legs to be handled easily, and is more sensitive. It is also easy to appreciate and visualise the anterior movement of the tibia and the end point is easy to detect. Nevertheless, it may still be influenced by muscle tone and soft tissue restraints.

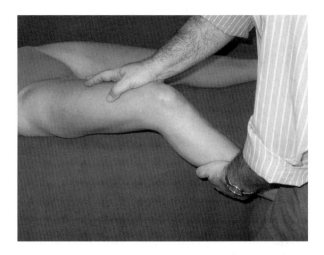

Fig 13.8 Determination of knee joint laxity using the Drop Leg Lachman test.

14 Ankle joint

ANATOMY

The ankle joint is a synovial hinge joint allowing adjustment of the line of gravity in the sagittal plane when standing and the provision of propulsion and restraint during gait.

The articulation is between the distal ends of the tibia and fibula proximally and the body of the talus distally (Fig. 14.1). The weight-bearing surfaces are the trochlear surfaces of the tibia and talus. The tibial trochlear surface is concave anteroposteriorly and convex transversely with a blunt sagittal ridge: the trochlear surface of the talus is reciprocally curved. Both surfaces are wider anteriorly than posteriorly. The tibial surface is continuous with the lateral surface of the medial malleolus, while the talar surface is continuous with those on the medial and lateral sides of the body.

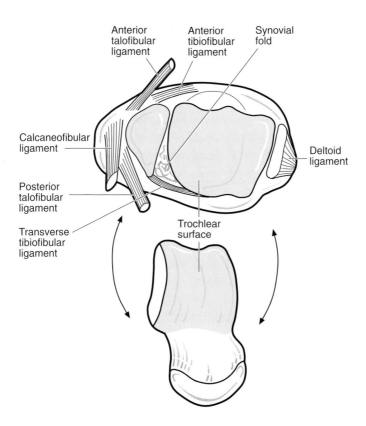

Fig 14.1 The articular surfaces of the ankle joint.

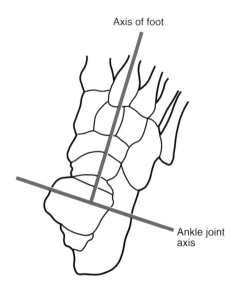

Axis of foot

Ankle joint
axis

Fig 14.2　The relation of the right ankle joint axis to the frontal plane.

The axis of the joint is horizontal but runs obliquely posterolaterally 20–25° from the frontal plane due to the outward rotation of the distal end of the tibia (Fig. 14.2). In plantarflexion the foot therefore moves downward and medially, while in dorsiflexion it moves upwards and laterally.

A fibrous capsule surrounds the joint, being thinner and weaker anteriorly and posteriorly than medially and laterally, where it is strengthened by collateral ligaments. Anteroposterior stability is provided by gravity keeping the trochlear surfaces in contact, while transverse stability depends on the two malleoli and collateral ligaments: maximum stability is achieved in full dorsiflexion.

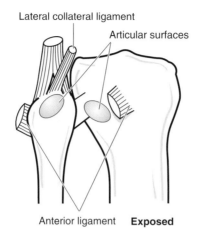

Lateral collateral ligament

Articular surfaces

(a)   Anterior ligament   **Exposed**

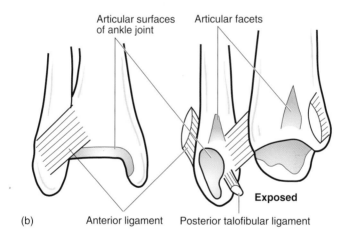

Articular surfaces
of ankle joint   Articular facets

(b)   Anterior ligament   Posterior talofibular ligament

                                             Exposed

Fig 14.3   The articular surfaces of the tibiofibular joints: (a) superior; (b) inferior.

The proximal and distal tibiofibular joints, although distinct from the ankle joint, subserve the function of the ankle joint. The plane synovial proximal tibiofibular joint is between the head of the fibula and the posteroinferolateral aspect of the lateral tibial condyle, while the fibrous distal joint is between the medial aspect of the distal fibula and the fibular notch of the tibia (Fig. 14.3). Movement occurs at both joints during plantarflexion and dorsiflexion.

RANGE OF MOVEMENT

Movement possible at the ankle joint is limited to plantarflexion (flexion) and dorsiflexion (extension), with the range of each being determined by the profiles of the articular surfaces. Plantarflexion and dorsiflexion cause a passive movement at both tibiofibular joints. In dorsiflexion the lateral malleolus moves laterally and superiorly, as well as rotating medially about its long axis: in dorsiflexion the converse occurs (Fig. 14.4).

Plantarflexion and dorsiflexion

The total range of active movement from full plantarflexion to full dorsi-flexion is 63° (Poulis and Soames), with 37° plantarflexion and 26° dorsi-flexion: Boone and Azen (1979), however, report a range of plantarflexion of 56°. Neonates have 59° dorsiflexion and 26° plantarflexion (Waugh *et al.*, 1983), while at age 2 the values are 41° and 62° respectively (Watanabe *et al.*, 1979). With increasing age the range of motion gradually decreases, with females having a greater range of both plantarflexion and dorsiflexion than males (Bell and Hoshizaki, 1981; Walker *et al.*, 1984).

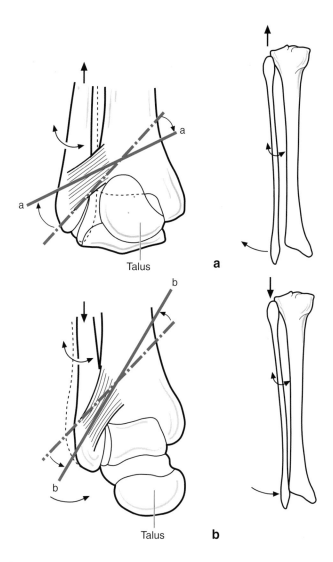

Talus

a

Talus

b

Fig 14.4 Movements of fibula accompanying movements at the ankle joint: (a) during dorsiflexion; (b) during plantarflexion.

Table 14.1 Ankle joint range of movement required for various activities	
Activity	Max range required
Gait on a level surface	15° dorsiflexion
	30° plantarflexion
Ascending stairs	25° dorsiflexion
	30° plantarflexion
Descending stairs	35° dorsiflexion
	30° plantarflexion
Putting on shoes	25° plantarflexion
Tying shoe laces	15° dorsiflexion

As the ankle joint is intimately associated with the restraint and propulsive phases of locomotor activities its functional range of motion must be adequate to avoid compromising these activities. However, there also needs to be sufficient range of motion to enable activities such as bending down to retrieve an object from the floor and putting on shoes. The ranges of motion associated with some common activities are given in Table 14.1.

Two accessory movements are possible at the ankle joint, these being longitudinal distraction and movement in an anterior–posterior direction. To elicit longitudinal distraction the subject lies supine and the calcaneus and head of the talus are gripped and pulled longitudinally in line with the tibia. For anterior–posterior movement the subject lies supine with the knee flexed and sole firmly pressed against the supporting surface. By gripping the distal ends of the tibia and fibula they can be moved anteriorly and posteriorly by pulling in the appropriate direction.

EVALUATION OF RANGE OF MOTION
Plantarflexion

With the subject sitting with the knee flexed to 90° and the foot in neutral abduction/adduction and pronation/supination, the tibia and fibula are stabilised to prevent knee movement and hip rotation (Fig. 14.5). The final resistance to movement is firm due to tension developed in the anterior joint capsule, the anterior components of the medial and lateral collateral ligaments and the extensor muscles crossing the joint: contact between the posterior talar tubercle and the posterior tibial margin may give a hard feel to the end point. To measure the degree of plantarflexion the centre of the goniometer is positioned over the lateral aspect of the lateral malleolus, with the proximal arm pointing towards the head of the fibula and the distal arm aligned with the fifth metatarsal.

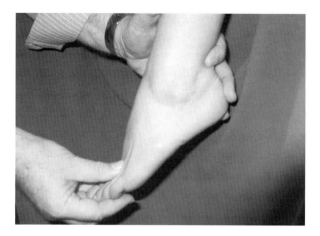

Fig 14.5 Determination of the range of plantarflexion at the ankle joint with the subject seated.

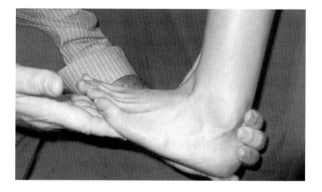

Fig 14.6 Determination of the range of dorsiflexion at the ankle joint with the subject seated.

Dorsiflexion

The subjects sits as for determining plantarflexion with the goniometer similarly aligned (Fig. 14.6). The final resistance to movement is again firm due to tension developed in the posterior joint capsule, the Achilles tendon and anterior components of the medial and lateral collateral ligaments.

15 Joints of the foot

INTRODUCTION

The foot comprises a series of joints which interact to provide support and adaptation to uneven surfaces during locomotor activities. The bones of the foot are arranged in longitudinal and transverse arches providing a structure strong enough to support body weight yet also flexible and resilient to absorb shocks transmitted to it. Maintenance of the arches depends on the integrity of the tarsal, tarsometatarsal and intertarsal joints proximally and metatarsophalangeal and interphalangeal joints distally.

The foot can be adducted and abducted about the long axis of the leg and pronated and supinated about its own long axis (Fig. 15.1). Because of the arrangement of the joints of the foot, particularly the subtalar and midtarsal joints, which both involve the talus, neither abduction/adduction nor pronation/supination can occur as pure movements. Adduction is always accompanied by supination giving inversion, while abduction is always accompanied by pronation giving eversion. An apparently pure movement of supination can be achieved by laterally rotating the leg at the knee to compensate for the accompanying adduction: similarly an apparently pure pronation can be achieved by medially rotating the leg at the knee to compensate for the accompanying abduction. When balancing on one leg, to enable full foot contact with the ground lateral rotation of the leg accompanies pronation of the forefoot: medial rotation accompanies supination of the forefoot under similar circumstances.

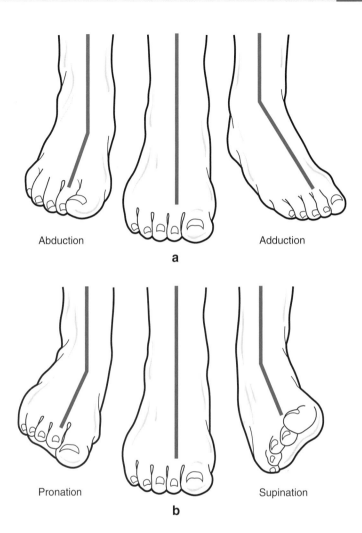

Abduction   Adduction

a

Pronation   Supination

b

Fig 15.1   (a) Abduction and adduction of the foot about the longitudinal axis of the leg; (b) pronation and supination of the foot about the longitudinal axis of the foot.

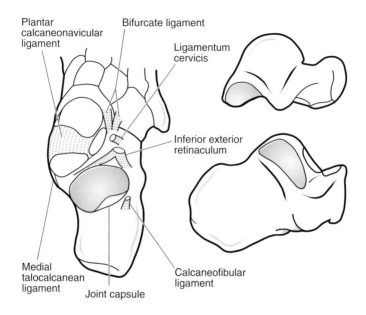

Plantar calcaneonavicular ligament

Bifurcate ligament

Ligamentum cervicis

Inferior exterior retinaculum

Medial talocalcanean ligament

Joint capsule

Calcaneofibular ligament

Fig 15.2 The articular surfaces of the subtalar joint.

SUBTALAR JOINT

The subtalar joint permits side-to-side adjustment of the line of gravity.

Anatomy

The subtalar joint is formed between the concave surface on the under-surface of the talus and the convex posterior facet on the upper surface of the calcaneus (Fig. 15.2). The oval calcaneal facet has its long axis running anterolaterally; it is this axis about which the facet is convex, being plane or concave about the other. The talar surface is reciprocally curved. Because of the shape of the articular surfaces there is limited mobility at the subtalar joint.

The joint is surrounded by a thin loose capsule reinforced by anterior, posterior, medial and lateral ligaments. The strong interosseous talocalcanean ligament acts as the fulcrum around which movements of the leg and foot occur, being continually subjected to twisting and stretching both at rest and during activity.

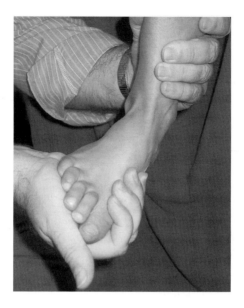

Fig 15.3 Determination of the range of pronation at the subtalar joint with the subject seated.

Evaluation of range of motion
Pronation

With the subject supine, the hip in neutral flexion/extension, abduction/adduction and medial/lateral rotation and the knee extended the foot is placed over the edge of the supporting surface (Fig. 15.3). The tibia and fibula are stabilised to prevent motion at the hip and knee and the heel turned laterally. The final resistance to movement is firm due to tension in the medial ligaments and tibialis posterior, or hard due to contact between the calcaneus and floor of the sinus tarsi. To measure the degree of pronation the centre of the goniometer is placed over the posterior aspect of the ankle midway between the two malleoli, with the proximal arm aligned with the midline of the back of the lower leg and the distal arm in line with the midline of the back of the calcaneus.

Alternatively the subject lies prone with the knee flexed to 90° and the ankle dorsiflexed until the soft tissues become taut (Fig. 15.4), the heel is then moved outward. The final resistance to movement is similar to above. The positioning of the goniometer is as described on page 149.

Supination

The subject is positioned as for measuring pronation, but the heel is turned medially (Fig. 15.5). The final resistance to movement is firm due to tension in the lateral and posterior ligaments, as well as the interosseous talocalcanean ligament. To measure the degree of supination the centre of the goniometer is placed over the posterior aspect of the ankle midway between the two malleoli, with the proximal arm aligned with the midline of the back of the lower leg and the distal arm in line with the midline of the back of the calcaneus.

Accessory movement

Accessory movement at the subtalar joint can be achieved by gripping and stabilising the talus hooking one hand in front of its anterior surface. Firm pressure applied to the back of the heel with the other hand causes the calcaneus to slide forwards on the talus.

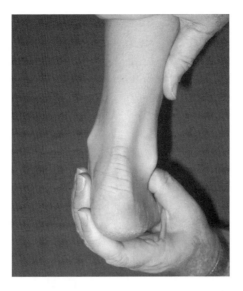

Fig 15.4 Determination of the range of pronation at the subtalar joint with the subject lying prone.

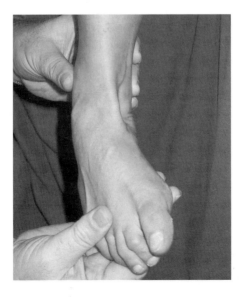

Fig 15.5 Determination of the range of supination at the subtalar joint with the subject seated.

MIDTARSAL JOINT

The midtarsal joint consists of two separate but linked joints, the talocal-caneonavicular and the calcaneocuboid joints, extending transversely across the foot (Fig. 15.6). The midtarsal joint enables the forefoot to move against the hindfoot.

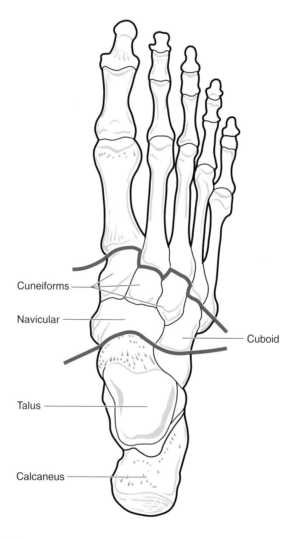

Cuneiforms

Navicular

Cuboid

Talus

Calcaneus

Fig 15.6 The midtarsal and tarsometatarsal joints of the foot.

Anatomy
Talocalcaneonavicular joint

A synovial joint between the head of the talus and the concavity of the posterior surface of the navicular, the superior surface of the sustentaculum tali and calcaneus and the plantar calcaneonavicular ligament (Fig. 15.7). A thin capsule, reinforced by the dorsal talonavicular and bifurcate ligaments, surrounds the joint.

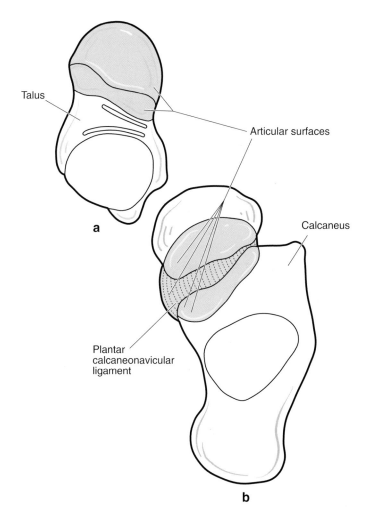

Talus

Articular surfaces

a

Calcaneus

Plantar calcaneonavicular ligament

b

Fig 15.7 The articular surfaces of the talocalcaneonavicular joint.

Calcaneocuboid joint

The articulation is between the anterior surface of the calcaneus and the posterior surface of the cuboid, both surfaces being gently undulating and quadrilateral in shape (Fig. 15.8). The upper part of the calcaneal surface is concave transversely and vertically, with the lower part being convex in both directions: the cuboid is reciprocally curved. There may be a medial flat extension of the cuboid for articulation with the navicular. A simple capsule surrounds the joint being reinforced by the dorsal and plantar calcaneocuboid ligaments.

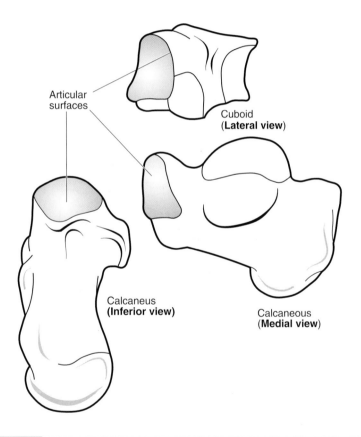

Articular surfaces

Cuboid
(**Lateral view**)

Calcaneus
(**Inferior view**)

Calcaneous
(**Medial view**)

Fig 15.8　The articular surfaces of the calcaneocuboid joint.

Evaluation of range of motion
Pronation

With the subject sitting with the knee flexed to 90° so that the leg is hanging over the edge of the supporting surface, the hip in neutral abduction/ adduction and medial/lateral rotation (Fig. 15.9). The calcaneus and talus are stabilised to prevent plantarflexion at the ankle and supination at the subtalar joint and the forefoot is turned laterally. The final resistance to movement is firm due to tension in the medial, dorsal and plantar ligaments and tibialis posterior. To measure the degree of pronation the centre of the goniometer is placed over the anterior aspect of the ankle just distal to a point midway between the malleoli, with the proximal arm aligned with the anterior midline of the lower leg and the distal arm aligned along the second metatarsal.

Alternatively the centre of the goniometer can be placed at the lateral aspect of the fifth metatarsal head, with the proximal arm parallel with the anterior midline of the lower leg and the distal arm aligned with the plantar surface of the metatarsal heads.

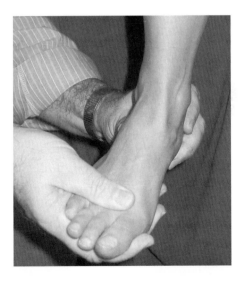

Fig 15.9 Determination of the range of pronation at the midtarsal joint with the subject seated.

Supination

The subject is positioned as for measuring pronation, but the forefoot is turned medially (Fig. 15.10). The final resistance to movement is firm due to tension in the lateral, dorsal and plantar ligaments and peroneus longus and brevis. To measure the degree of supination the centre of the goniometer is placed over the anterior aspect of the ankle just distal to a point midway between the malleoli, with the proximal arm aligned with the anterior midline of the lower leg and the distal arm aligned along the second metatarsal.

Alternatively the centre of the goniometer can be placed at the medial aspect of the first metatarsal head, with the proximal arm parallel to the anterior midline of the leg and the distal arm aligned with the plantar surfaces of the metatarsal heads.

Accessory movement

Accessory movement at the calcaneocuboid joint is achieved by gripping the calcaneus firmly with one hand and the cuboid with the other: holding the calcaneus still the cuboid can slide up and down against it.

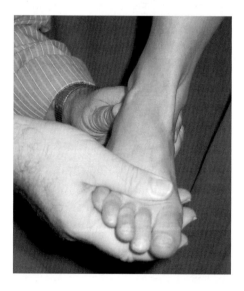

Fig 15.10 Determination of the range of supination at the midtarsal joint with the subject seated.

Range of movement

The range of movement at the subtalar and midtarsal joints are best considered together since it is difficult to determine movement at each individually: the combined movement being eversion and inversion. Boone and Azen (1979) report a total range of pronation/supination of 58°, being 21° pronation and 37° supination. Roaas and Andersson (1982) give a slightly smaller total range (56°), but consider the ranges of pronation and supination to be equal.

Evaluation of the range of motion of eversion and inversion

Eversion

With the subject sitting with the knee flexed to 90° and the leg hanging over the edge of the supporting surface, the hip in neutral abduction/adduction and medial/lateral rotation and the foot everted (Fig. 15.11). The tibia and fibula are stabilised to prevent lateral rotation and flexion at the knee and medial rotation and adduction at the hip. The final resistance to movement

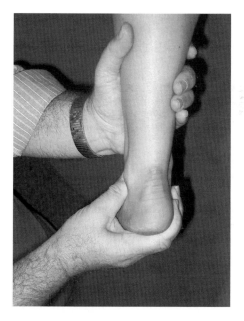

Fig 15.11   Determination of the range of eversion of the foot with the subject seated.

is firm due to tension in the medial, dorsal and plantar ligaments and tibialis posterior. However, if there is contact between the calcaneus and floor of the sinus tarsi the final resistance will be hard. To measure the degree of eversion the centre of the goniometer is placed over the anterior ankle midway between the malleoli, with the proximal arm directed towards the tibial tuberosity and the distal arm aligned along the second metatarsal.

Inversion

The subject is positioned as for determining eversion. The tibia and fibula are stabilised to prevent medial rotation and extension at the knee and lateral rotation and abduction at the hip and the foot inverted (Fig. 15.12). The final resistance to movement is firm due to tension in anterior, posterior, lateral, dorsal and plantar ligaments and peroneus longus and brevis. To measure the degree of inversion the centre of the goniometer is placed over the anterior ankle midway between the malleoli, with the proximal arm directed towards the tibial tuberosity and the distal arm aligned along the second metatarsal.

TARSOMETATARSAL JOINTS

These plane synovial overlapping joints are between the three cuneiforms and cuboid posteriorly and the bases of the five metatarsals anteriorly. The joint line is irregular and arched; however, the joints are fairly mobile, contributing to the pronation and supination of the forefoot: the joint line runs from anteromedial to posterolateral (Fig. 15.6). The first metatarsal articulates with the medial cuneiform forming a separate joint medially. The second metatarsal is held in a mortise formed by the three cuneiforms, while the third articulates with lateral cuneiform; together they form the intermediate joint. The lateral joint cavity is formed by the fourth metatarsal which articulates mainly with the cuboid but also the lateral cuneiform, and the fifth metatarsal with the cuboid. All joints are surrounded by capsules which are reinforced by dorsal, plantar and interosseous tarsometatarsal ligaments. Small plane intermetatarsal joints are formed between the adjacent surfaces of the lateral four metatarsals.

Because of the obliquity of the axis about which flexion and extension take place, plantarflexion at the joints is accompanied by adduction while abduction accompanies dorsiflexion. The obliquity of the first tarsometatarsal joint means that plantarflexion of the first metatarsal is accompanied by 15° adduction. The mobility of the first metatarsal is necessary to enable the foot to adapt to the ground during inversion and eversion, particularly when walking on uneven surfaces.

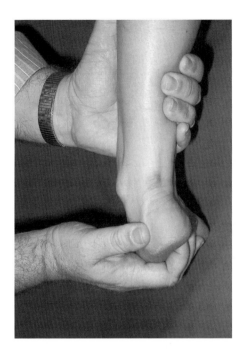

Fig 15.12 Determination of the range of inversion of the foot with the subject seated.

Accessory movements

Accessory movements between adjacent bones is achieved by holding one bone steady and moving the other. The largest movement possible is between the base of the fifth metatarsal and the cuboid.

METATARSOPHALANGEAL JOINTS
Anatomy

The condyloid metatarsophalangeal joints are between the rounded meta-tarsal heads and the cupped base of the proximal phalanx (Fig. 15.13). The plantar articular surface of the metatarsal head is more extensive than the dorsal, enabling a greater range of plantarflexion at the joint. During dorsiflexion the toes spread apart and become inclined laterally, while in plantarflexion they are pulled together. Each joint is surrounded by a loose capsule reinforced laterally by strong collateral ligaments, dorsally by the extensor expansion and on their plantar aspect by the plantar ligament. Each joint permits flexion–extension and adduction–abduction.

Range of movement

There appear to be few studies that have determined the range of movement of the metatarsophalangeal joint for either the hallux or the other toes. However, Shereff *et al.* (1986) reported a total range of 110° for the hallux, of which the majority is dorsiflexion. Observation suggests that the remaining toes have a total range of movement between 80° medially and 40° laterally, again with the majority of movement being dorsiflexion. Because of the immobility of the second metatarsal abduction/adduction takes place about the axis of the second toe.

Evaluating the range of motion
Plantarflexion

With the subject lying supine or sitting with the foot extending over the edge of the supporting surface (Fig. 15.14), the ankle, foot, metatarsophalangeal and interphalangeal joints should be in neutral dorsiflexion/plantarflexion, neutral inversion/eversion, abduction/adduction and dorsiflexion/plantarflexion respectively. If the ankle and interphalangeal joints are plantarflexed movement is restricted due to tension in the extensor muscles. The metatarsal is stabilised to prevent ankle plantarflexion and inversion or eversion of the foot. The remaining toes should not be held in extension as tension in the deep transverse metatarsal ligament will also restrict movement. The final resistance is firm due to tension in the dorsal joint capsule and collateral ligaments.

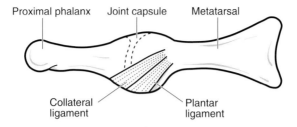

Proximal phalanx   Joint capsule   Metatarsal

Collateral
ligament

Plantar
ligament

Fig 15.13 The anatomy of the metatarsophalangeal joints.

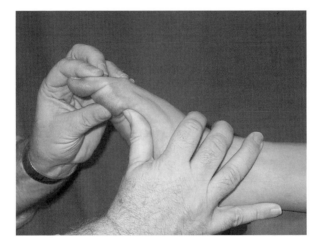

Fig 15.14 Determination of the range of plantarflexion at the first metatarsophalangeal joint.

Hallux

To measure the degree of plantarflexion of the hallux the centre of the goniometer is placed over the medial aspect of the metatarsophalangeal joint, with the proximal arm along the medial midline of the first metatarsal and the distal arm aligned with the medial midline of the proximal phalanx.

Lesser toes

To measure the degree of plantarflexion of the remaining toes the centre of the goniometer is placed over the dorsal aspect of the metatarsophalangeal joint, with the proximal arm over the dorsal midline of the metatarsal and the distal arm aligned with the dorsal midline of the proximal phalanx.

Dorsiflexion

The subject is positioned as for plantarflexion. If the ankle and interphalangeal joints are dorsiflexed movement is restricted due to tension in the flexor muscles: if the interphalangeal joints are in extreme flexion tension in the lumbricals and interosseii may also restrict movement (Fig. 15.15). The metatarsal is stabilised to prevent ankle dorsiflexion and inversion or eversion of the foot. The final resistance to movement is firm due to tension in the plantar joint capsule and the plantar ligament.

Hallux

To measure the degree of dorsiflexion of the hallux the centre of the goniometer is placed over the medial aspect of the metatarsophalangeal joint, with the proximal arm along the medial midline of the first metatarsal and the distal arm aligned with the medial midline of the proximal phalanx.

Lesser toes

To measure the degree of dorsiflexion of the remaining toes the centre of the goniometer is placed over the dorsal aspect of the metatarsophalangeal joint, with the proximal arm over the dorsal midline of the metatarsal and the distal arm aligned with the dorsal midline of the proximal phalanx.

Abduction

With the subject lying supine or sitting with the foot in neutral inversion/eversion and the metatarsophalangeal and interphalangeal joints in neutral dorsiflexion/plantarflexion the first, third, fourth and fifth toes can be moved away from the second (Fig. 15.16). The metatarsal is stabilised to prevent inversion or eversion. The final resistance to movement

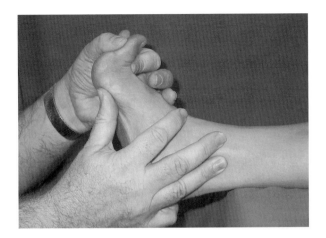

Fig 15.15 Determination of the range of dorsiflexion at the first metatarsophalangeal joint.

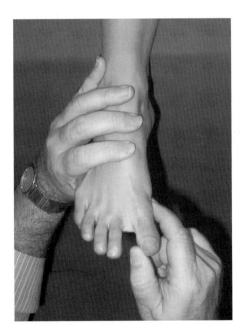

Fig 15.16 Determination of the range of abduction at the first metatarsophalangeal joint.

is firm due to tension in the joint capsule, collateral ligaments and fascia in the web spaces. To measure the degree of abduction the centre of the goniometer is placed over the dorsal aspect of the metatarsophalangeal joint, with the proximal arm along the dorsal midline of the metatarsal and the dorsal arm aligned with the dorsal midline of the proximal phalanx.

Accessory movments

Accessory movements are possible between the head of the metatarsal and the base of the proximal phalanx. Gripping the head of the metatarsal the proximal phalanx can be slid up and down as well as rotated against it.

INTERPHALANGEAL JOINTS
Anatomy

The joints are between the head of one phalanx and the base of the distal phalanx in series (Fig. 15.17). The articular surface of the metatarsal head is pulley-shaped appearing as a double convexity, with a double concavity on the base of the more distal phalanx. Each joint is surrounded by a capsule, which is reinforced (or replaced) by the collateral ligaments at the sides, dorsally by the extensor expansion and on its plantar surface by the plantar ligament. The distal interphalangeal joint of the little toe is often obliterated.

Range of movement

Due to the shape of the articular surfaces the interphalangeal joints only permit plantarflexion and dorsiflexion. The American Academy of Orthopaedic Surgeons (1994) report that the range of motion for the hallux is 45° plantarflexion and 70° dorsiflexion. For the lesser toes the ranges of motion at the proximal interphalangeal joint are 35° and 40° respectively, and for the distal interphalangeal joint 60° and 40° respectively.

Evaluation of range of motion
Dorsiflexion of the proximal interphalangeal joint

With the subject lying supine or sitting with the ankle in neutral dorsiflexion/plantarflexion and the foot in neutral inversion/eversion (Fig. 15.18), the metatarsophalangeal joint is in neutral dorsiflexion/plantarflexion and abduction/adduction. If the ankle and metatarsophalangeal joints are plantarflexed motion is restricted due to tension in the extensor muscles; if the metatarsophalangeal joint is in full dorsiflexion tension in the lumbrical and interosseii muscles may also limit motion.

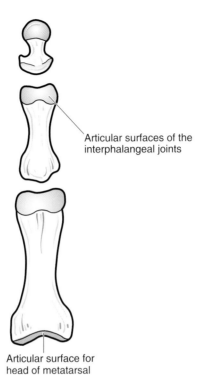

Articular surfaces of the
interphalangeal joints

Articular surface for
head of metatarsal

Fig 15.17 The articular surfaces of the interphalangeal joints.

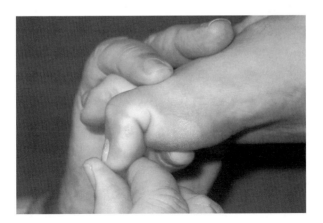

Fig 15.18 Determination of the range of plantarflexion at the
interphalangeal of the first toe.

The metatarsal and proximal phalanx are stabilised to prevent movement at the ankle or inversion/eversion of the foot. Movement at the metatarso-phalangeal joint should also be avoided. The final resistance to movement is soft due to compression of soft tissue between the plantar surfaces; however, it may be firm due to tension in the dorsal joint capsule and collateral ligaments.

Hallux

To measure the degree of dorsiflexion the centre of the goniometer is placed over the medial aspect of the interphalangeal joint, with the proximal arm along the medial midline of the proximal phalanx and the distal arm aligned along the medial midline of the distal phalanx.

Lesser toes

To measure the degree of dorsiflexion the centre of the goniometer is placed over the dorsal aspect of the joint being tested, with the proximal arm over the dorsal midline of the proximal phalanx and the distal arm over the dorsal midline of the intermediate phalanx.

Plantarflexion of the proximal interphalangeal joint

The subject is positioned as for determining dorsiflexion. If the ankle and metatarsophalangeal joints are dorsiflexed motion is limited by tension in the flexor muscles. The final resistance to movement is firm due to tension in the plantar joint capsule and plantar ligament.

Hallux

To measure the degree of plantarflexion the centre of the goniometer is placed over the medial aspect of the interphalangeal joint, with the proximal arm along the medial midline of the proximal phalanx and the distal arm aligned along the medial midline of the distal phalanx.

Lesser toes

To measure the degree of plantarflexion the centre of the goniometer is placed over the dorsal aspect of the joint being tested, with the proximal arm over the dorsal midline of the proximal phalanx and the distal arm over the dorsal midline of the middle phalanx.

Plantarflexion of the distal interphalangeal joints

With the subject lying supine or sitting with the ankle and foot in neutral dorsiflexion/plantarflexion and inversion/eversion respectively, the metatarsophalangeal and proximal interphalangeal joints are also in neutral. If the ankle, metatarsophalangeal and proximal interphalangeal joints are plantarflexed motion is restricted by tension in the extensor muscles. If the metatarsophalangeal and proximal interphalangeal joints are in full extension additional tension in the oblique retinacular ligament also restricts movement. The metatarsal, proximal and middle phalanx are stabilised to prevent movement at the ankle or inversion/eversion of the foot: movement at the metatarsophalangeal and proximal interphalangeal joints must also be prevented. The final resistance to movement is firm due to tension in the dorsal joint capsule, collateral and oblique retinacular ligaments. To measure the degree of plantarflexion the centre of the goniometer is placed over the dorsal aspect of the joint, with the proximal arm along the dorsal midline of the middle phalanx and the distal arm over the dorsal midline of the distal phalanx.

Dorsiflexion of the distal interphalangeal joint

The subject is positioned as for determining dorsiflexion. If the ankle, metatarsophalangeal and proximal interphalangeal joints are dorsiflexed movement is limited due to tension in the flexor muscles, lumbricals and interosseii. The metatarsal, proximal and middle phalanx are stabilised to prevent movement at the ankle or inversion/eversion of the foot: movement at the metatarsophalangeal and proximal interphalangeal joints must also be prevented. The final resistance to movement is firm due to tension in the plantar joint capsule and plantar ligament. To measure the degree of plantarflexion the centre of the goniometer is placed over the dorsal aspect of the joint, with the proximal arm along the dorsal midline of the middle phalanx and the distal arm over the dorsal midline of the distal phalanx.

Accessory movements

Accessory movements are possible between the head of the most proximal phalanx and the base of the more distal phalanx. Gripping the head of the proximal phalanx the more distal phalanx can be slid up and down against it.

16 Vertebral column

INTRODUCTION

The vertebral column is the composite articulation of 24 contiguous vertebrae between their bodies (secondary cartilaginous joints) and articular processes (synovial joints) (Fig. 16.1): the articulations between C1 and C2 (atlantoaxial joint) do not follow this pattern. The column articulates with the skull at the occipital condyles (atlanto-occipital joint) and the sacrum by the lumbosacral joint (page 104). Individual articulations have a limited range of movement, determined partly by the shape and orientation of the articular processes and partly by the degree of hydration of the individual intervertebral discs. In the lumbar and cervical regions where the discs are thick in relation to the vertebral bodies the range of movement between adjacent vertebrae is increased.

The basic movements of the vertebral column are flexion (forward bending) and extension (backward bending) about a transverse axis with a total range of 270°, lateral flexion (bending) about an anteroposterior axis with a total range of 100°, and axial rotation about a vertical axis with a total range of 110°. All movements are possible in each region of the vertebral column, although their magnitude may be extremely small. Lateral flexion and rotation are linked with neither being possible independently.

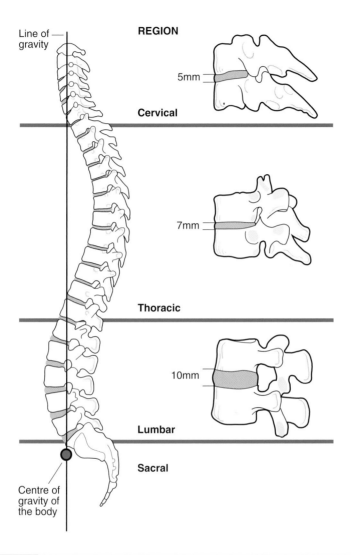

Line of gravity

REGION

5mm

Cervical

7mm

Thoracic

10mm

Lumbar

Sacral

Centre of gravity of the body

Fig 16.1 The adult vertebral column showing the curvatures (left hand side) and articulations between the vertebral bodies and articular facets (right hand side).

ANATOMY

Individual vertebrae consist of a body anteriorly and a neural arch posteriorly (Fig. 16.2). The superior and inferior surfaces of the bodies of C3 to L5 are covered with hyaline cartilage, with adjacent surfaces being separated by a fibrocartilaginous intervertebral disc: only the inferior surface of C2 has a covering of hyaline cartilage. In the cervical region the discs do not extend the full width of the bodies: small synovial joints (uncovertebral joints) are formed between the adjacent lateral parts of adjacent bodies (Fig. 16.3). These joints help to control movement of the cervical spine.

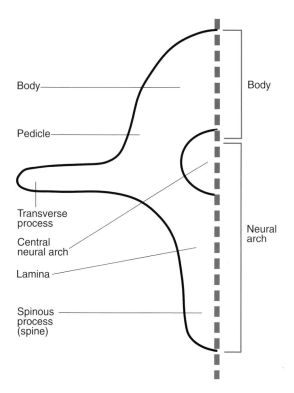

Body

Body

Pedicle

Neural
arch

Transverse
process

Central
neural arch

Lamina

Spinous
process
(spine)

Fig 16.2 Plan of a typical vertebra.

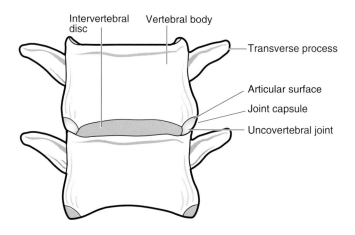

Intervertebral
disc

Vertebral body

Transverse process

Articular surface

Joint capsule

Uncovertebral joint

Fig 16.3 The uncovertebral joints associated with cervical vertebra.

The neural arches are united by synovial joints (zygapophyseal joints), the shape and orientation of which differ in each region (Fig. 16.4). A thin lax fibrous capsule surrounds each joint: accessory ligaments help to stabilise and unite the neural arches. The ligamentum flavum extends between the adjacent laminae between C1/C2 and L4/L5; the supraspinous ligament connects the tips of adjacent spinous processes, in the cervical region it is replaced by the ligamentum nuchae running from C7 to the external occipital protuberance; thin membranous interspinous ligaments unite adjacent vertebral spines, being stronger in the lumbar region; the intertransverse ligaments are only present in the lumbar region, often being replaced by muscles in the upper part of the vertebral column.

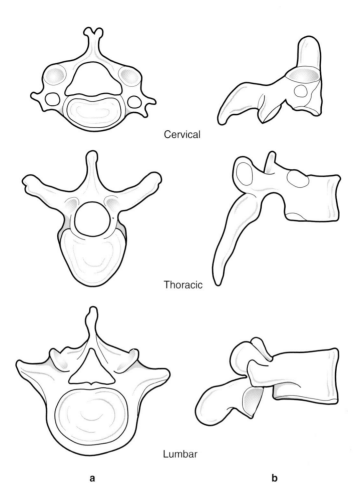

Cervical

Thoracic

Lumbar

a   b

Fig 16.4 The orientation of the articular facets of the zygapophyseal joints in the cervical, thoracic and lumbar regions of the vertebral column: (a) superior view; (b) lateral view.

CERVICAL REGION

Because of the specialised nature of C1 and C2 the cervical spine is usually considered to consist of two segments: the sub-occipital and the lower cervical segments. The sub-occipital segment comprises the atlanto-occipital and atlantoaxial joints, while the lower cervical segment is that region between C2 and C7.

Anatomy
Sub-occipital segment

Each synovial atlanto-occipital articulation is between a concave oval facet on the upper surface of the lateral mass of the atlas (C1) and the reciprocally curved convex occipital condyle: the two joints are symmetrical and act as a single functional unit. The long axes of the joints pass obliquely to converge in the midline anterior to the anterior arch of the atlas.

The atlantoaxial articulations comprise bilateral synovial joints between the convex oval facets on the superior process of the axis (C2) and concave facets on the atlas, and two median synovial joints formed between the dens and the anterior arch and transverse ligament of the atlas. Alar ligaments pass obliquely superolaterally from the apex of the dens to the medial side of each occipital condyle, while the apical ligament of the dens attaches to the anterior margin of the foramen magnum.

Lower cervical segment

The articulation between adjacent vertebrae is by flat oval facets on the superior and inferior projections from the body: the facets lie in an oblique plane, with the obliquity increasing from above downwards.

Range of movement

Although the two segments are functionally distinct they are complementary, enabling flexion–extension, lateral flexion and axial rotation. Because of the relative thickness of cervical intervertebral discs, as well as the shape and orientation of the articular facets, movement associated with the lower cervical segment is quite extensive in all three planes. Flexion–extension occurs in the sagittal plane about a mediolateral axis, lateral flexion in the frontal plane about an anteroposterior axis, and axial rotation in the transverse plane about a vertical axis. The range of movement, where appropriate, is given for each segment, although in the evaluation of the range of motion no distinction between the segments is made.

Flexion and extension

The range of flexion and extension in the lower cervical segment is approximately 110°, the least movement is between C7 and T1, with that in the sub-occipital segment being 20–25°, giving a total range of cervical movement of 135° (AAOS, 1994). This is in close agreement with the range of 130° reported by Capuano-Pucci *et al.* (1991). In both sexes up to age 20 the range of flexion is 64° and extension 85° (Youdas *et al.*, 1992), decreasing to 36° flexion and 50° extension by age 90 (Youdas *et al.*, 1992). The loss of motion is on average 3° with each 10-year increase in age for flexion and 5° for extension in both sexes; however, over age 30 females tend to have greater ranges of movement than males.

Lateral flexion

The total range of lateral flexion is similar on the right and left sides, being 45° (AAOS, 1994), with 40° occurring in the lower cervical segment. After age 40 lateral flexion gradually decreases so that by age 90 it is 24° (Youdas *et al.*, 1992). Again over age 30 females have a slightly greater range of motion.

Rotation

There is no difference in the total range of rotation to the right or left sides, being 70° (Youdas *et al.*, 1992), of which 15° occurs at the sub-occipital segment. The majority of the sub-occipital motion is at the atlantoaxial joint, with C1 and the head moving as a single unit. Because of the obliquity of the lateral atlantoaxial joint surfaces and convexity of the facets, sub-occipital rotation can be increased by tilting the head backwards and to the opposite side. Beyond age 30 rotation gradually decreases to 50° at age 90 (Youdas *et al.*, 1992), with females having a greater range in later years than males.

Accessory movements

Accessory movements are present in the cervical joints, being either general or local: they should not be attempted without specific training and then with care and caution. Traction of the cervical spine is a general movement affecting the neck as a whole. Several millimetres elongation can be achieved producing distraction of the discs and facet joints; there is negligible movement between C2 and the base of the skull. A side-to-side movement can be achieved by moving the head to the right or left when it is in the upright position. Local accessory movement can be produced by applying pressure to the spines, transverse or articular processes of individual vertebrae.

Evaluation of range of motion
Flexion

With the subject seated and the pectoral girdle supported against a chair back to prevent thoracic or lumbar flexion or extension during the movement, the head is placed in neutral flexion/extension, lateral flexion and rotation. The centre of the goniometer is placed over the external auditory meatus with one arm vertical (a small plumb line attached to the proximal arm helps to achieve this) and the other aligned with the base of the nares: if a tongue depressor is held between the teeth the distal arm can be aligned parallel with the tongue depressor. Pressure is applied to the back of the head to maintain flexion, while gently pulling the chin towards the chest: the mouth should remain closed (Fig. 16.5). Care must be taken to prevent thoracic and/or lumbar flexion.

Extension

From the same starting position and goniometer alignment for flexion the head is tilted backwards by applying pressure to the chin; rotation and lateral flexion of the neck are prevented by holding the chin (Fig. 16.6). Thoracic and/or lumbar extension are prevented by the presence of the chair back.

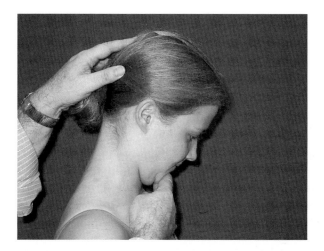

Fig 16.5 Determination of the range of flexion of the cervical spine.

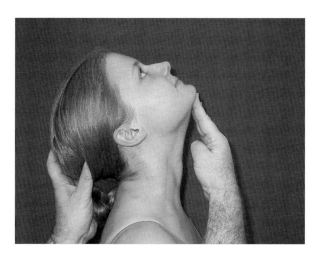

Fig 16.6 Determination of the range of extension of the cervical spine.

An alternative method of estimating the total range of cervical motion is to use a tape measure to measure the distance between the chin and sternal notch in full flexion and full extension. However, this does not provide an angular measure of flexion–extension.

Lateral flexion

With the subject seated and the thoracic and lumbar spine supported by a chair back the head is placed in neutral flexion/extension, rotation and lateral flexion. The centre of the goniometer is placed over the spinous process of C7 with one arm aligned with the spinous processes of the thoracic vertebrae and the other aligned with the external occipital protuberance. With one hand placed on the opposite shoulder to prevent lateral flexion of the thoracic and lumbar spine the cervical spine is maintained in lateral flexion by pulling the head laterally (Fig. 16.7).

Alternatively, an estimate of lateral flexion can be achieved by measuring the distance between the mastoid process and acromion using a tape measure.

Rotation

With the subject seated and the thoracic and lumbar spine supported the head is placed in neutral flexion/extension, lateral flexion and rotation. The centre of the goniometer is placed over the centre of the vertex of the head with one arm parallel to a line passing between the acromion processes and the other aligned with the tip of the nose. With one hand placed on the opposite shoulder to prevent rotation of the thoracic and lumbar spine neck rotation is maintained by rotating the head while preventing cervical flexion/extension and lateral flexion (Fig. 16.8).

Alternatively, an estimate of rotation can be achieved by measuring the distance between the chin and acromion process using a tape measure.

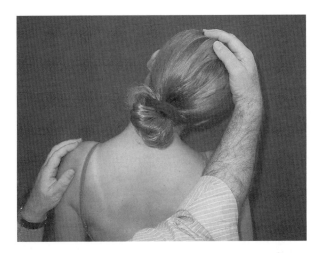

Fig 16.7 Determination of the range of lateral flexion of the cervical spine.

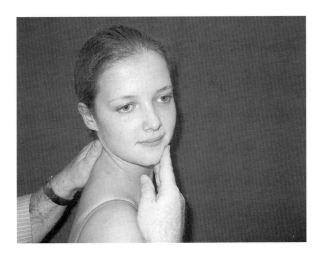

Fig 16.8 Determination of the range of rotation of the cervical spine.

THORACIC AND LUMBAR REGIONS
Anatomy

The articular processes of thoracic vertebrae project almost vertically superiorly and inferiorly from the base of the transverse process. The facets on the superior process are gently concave transversely, being flat from above down and face posteriorly, while those on the inferior process are reciprocally curved and face anteriorly. The zygapophyseal joints so formed lie on the arc of a circle whose centre lies either within the body of the vertebrae or just anterior to it. The bodies and transverse processes of thoracic vertebrae also carry facets for articulation of the ribs.

The articular processes of lumbar vertebrae project superiorly and inferiorly from the junction of the pedicles and laminae. The facets on the superior processes are concave transversely, flat vertically and face posteromedially, while those on the inferior processes are reciprocally curved and face anterolaterally. The inferior facets of L5 are flatter, set more widely apart and face mainly forward for articulation with the sacrum.

Range of movement

The intervertebral discs of the thoracic region are relatively thin with respect to the vertebral bodies, which together with the ribs and sternum tend to limit movement; nevertheless flexion, extension, lateral flexion and rotation are all permitted. Because the inferior processes of T12, or occasionally T11 and thus those on T12, resemble lumbar facets movements of the thoracolumbar junction are similar to those between lumbar vertebrae. The thoracic region of the spine is, in general, less flexible than the cervical.

The intervertebral discs in the lumbar region are relatively thick; however, the orientation of the articular processes tends to confer stability to this region. Nevertheless flexion, extension and lateral flexion are free with rotation being restricted.

Although the two regions are structurally and functionally distinct the movements possible in each are complementary. Consequently the total range of movement for the thoracolumbar spine is given; however, where appropriate the separate ranges for each region are given. Evaluation of the ranges of movement considers both regions together.

Flexion and extension

The total range of flexion and extension may be as much as 135°; however, the AAOS (1994) give a value of 110°, with flexion exceeding extension. Flexion of the thoracic spine is approximately half that of the lumbar spine due to the presence of the ribs (30° and 55° respectively), while extension is two-thirds that in the lumbar region (20° and 30° respectively). Males have a greater range of both flexion (Macrae and Wright, 1969) and extension (Moll *et al.*, 1972) than females at all ages, with both flexion and extension decreasing with age (Fitzgerald *et al.*, 1983); the change in extension being greater than that for flexion (Sughara *et al.*, 1981).

Lateral flexion

The total range of lateral flexion is 55° to each side with that in the thoracic and lumbar regions being similar, 25° and 30° respectively. Between the ages of 30 and 80 lateral flexion has been observed to decrease by 50% (Fitzgerald *et al.*, 1983).

Rotation

The total range of rotation to each side is 40°, the majority (35°) being associated with the thoracic region: it is greatest in the mid-thoracic region. A 50% reduction in range has been observed between the ages of 30 and 80 (Fitzgerald *et al.*, 1983).

The age-related changes reported for all movements are consistent with the age-related changes reported in intervertebral discs.

Accessory movements

Accessory movements in the thoracic region are small, but can be demonstrated by applying local pressure over the spinous process to produce a rocking of the vertebral body, while when applied over the base of the transverse process produces separation of the zygapophyseal joint. In the lumbar region rocking of the vertebral body is achieved by applying pressure to one side of the spinous process, while forward gliding of the vertebra is achieved by applying pressure to the spinous or mamillary process.

Evaluation of range of motion

The angular measurement of flexion and extension is difficult without using specialised goniometers. The easiest method for obtaining an estimate of the ranges of flexion and extension is with a tape measure.

Flexion

With the subject standing with the feet slightly apart and the spine in neutral lateral flexion and rotation the pelvis is stabilised to prevent anterior tilting by placing one hand over the anterior aspect of the pelvis. With one end of the tape placed over the spinous process of S1 and the other over the spinous process of C7 a reading is taken when standing erect: a second reading is taken in full flexion (Fig. 16.9). The difference in readings is a measure of thoracolumbar flexion: a difference of 10 cm is considered to be normal (AAOS, 1994). By having the ends of the tape over the spinous processes of T12 and C7, and S1 and T12 the contribution to the total movement made by the thoracic and lumbar spines can be determined.

An alternative method is the Modified Schober Technique in which the lumbosacral junction is marked, with a second mark made 10 cm above the first and a third 5 cm above the second. The tape is aligned between the top and bottom marks and readings taken with the subject erect and in full flexion; the range of flexion is the difference between the initial 15 cm and length when flexed. This technique is, however, essentially a measure of lumbar flexion.

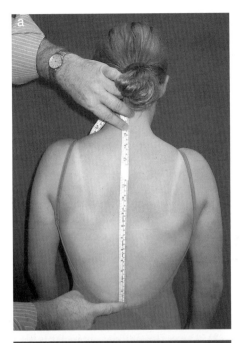

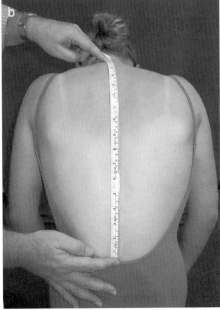

Fig 16.9 Determination of the range of flexion of the thoracic and lumbar spine: (a) spine in neutral; (b) spine flexed.

Extension

With the subject in the same initial posture posterior tilting of the pelvis is prevented by placing one hand over the anterior aspect of the pelvis and the other over the posterior pelvis. Place the ends of the tape over the spinous processes of S1 and C7 (Fig. 16.10). The difference in readings between the erect position and full extension is an indication of thoracolumbar extension. The measurements can be taken with the subject either prone or when lying on the side: it is easier to stabilise the pelvis with the subject lying prone.

Alternatively, the Modified Schober Technique can be used as for flexion, in which case the subject should be instructed to place their hands on the buttocks and bend backwards as far as possible. The difference in readings between the initial 15 cm and that observed when bending backwards is an indication of (lumbar) extension.

Lateral flexion

With the subject standing with the feet slightly apart and the spine in neutral flexion/extension and rotation the pelvis is stabilised to prevent lateral tilting by placing one hand over the opposite iliac crest to the direction of bending (Fig. 16.11). The centre of the goniometer is placed over the posterior aspect of the S1 spinous process, with the proximal arm aligned with the spinous process of C7 and the distal arm aligned perpendicular to the ground. During the movement the proximal arm is kept aligned with C7 and not the vertebral column since the lower thoracic and lumbar spine becomes convex to the side of flexion.

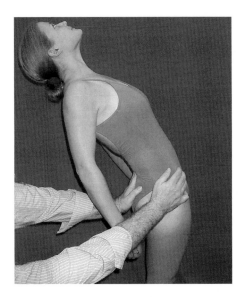

Fig 16.10 Determination of the range of extension of the thoracic and lumbar spine.

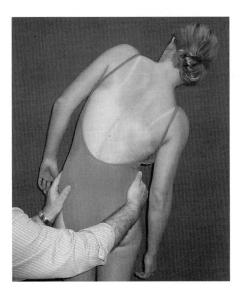

Fig 16.11 Determination of the range of lateral flexion of the thoracic and lumbar spine.

An alternative method is to measure the difference in distance between the tip of the middle finger and the floor between standing erect and lateral flexion, ensuring that there is no lateral tilting of the pelvis, the knees are extended and the feet remain flat on the floor.

Rotation

With the subject seated comfortably erect on a stool with the feet on the floor and the spine in neutral flexion/extension and lateral bending the hands are placed on both iliac crests to prevent pelvic rotation (Fig. 16.12). The centre of the goniometer is placed over the centre of the vertex of the head with one arm parallel to a line passing between the acromion processes and the other aligned parallel to a line passing through the iliac tubercles.

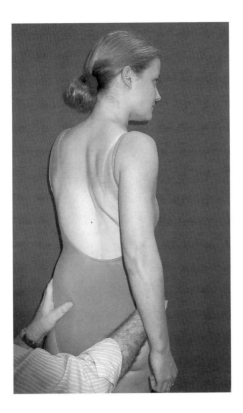

Fig 16.12 Determination of the range of rotation of the thoracic and lumbar spine.

17 Temporomandibular joint

ANATOMY

The temporomandibular joint is a synovial condyloid joint between the mandibular fossa of the temporal bone on the base of the skull and the condyle (head) of the mandible, divided into two distinct parts by a complete intra-articular disc. The mandibular fossa is oval with a wide concave mediolateral surface and a concavoconvex (from behind forwards) anteroposterior surface (Fig. 17.1). The mandibular condyle is smaller than the mandibular fossa and has its long axis running posteromedially, making an angle with the frontal plane of 30°. The intra-articular disc moulds itself between the articular surfaces and enables different movements to occur in each of the two parts of the joint.

A strong, but thin and loose, fibrous capsule surrounds the joint being reinforced laterally by the lateral ligament. The accessory sphenomandibular and stylomandibular ligaments are important in controlling and limiting movement at the joint.

RANGE OF MOVEMENT

Different movements occur in each of the two parts of the joint: protraction and retraction takes place in the upper compartment and elevation and depression in the lower, while side-to-side movements take place in both compartments.

Protraction and retraction

During protraction the head of the mandible and disc glide forward together in the mandibular fossa as far as the articular eminence: the opposite movement is retraction. This movement occurs in the upper compartment of the joint. The average range of movement for protraction is 6–9 mm (Friedman and Weisberg, 1982), while that for retraction is 3–4 mm.

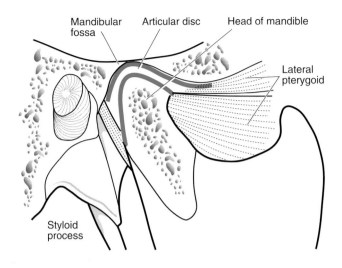

Fig 17.1 The articular surfaces of the temporomandibular joint: sagittal section.

Elevation and depression

Elevation and depression involve rotation of the head of the mandible against the disc, and takes place in the lower compartment of the joint. The mouth should be capable of opening sufficiently to enable two or three flexed proximal interphalangeal joints to be inserted into the opening. The distance required for opening ranges from 35–50 mm.

Lateral deviation

Lateral deviation accompanies side-to-side movement of the mandible, the two sides of the mandible moving in opposite directions: one side is elevated and protracted while the other is depressed and retracted. Lateral deviation has a range of 10–12 mm.

Accessory movements

Lateral pressure applied to the head of the mandible causes it to move transversely within the mandibular fossa, while pressure applied from behind the ear to the back of the condyle results in forward movement of the condyle.

EVALUATION OF RANGE OF MOVEMENT
Protraction

With the subject seated, the head and neck are stabilised to prevent flexion, extension, lateral flexion and rotation of the cervical spine, the mandible is protracted (Fig. 17.2). A marked plastic rule or one arm of a goniometer is placed in the mouth and the distance between the upper and lower incisors measured.

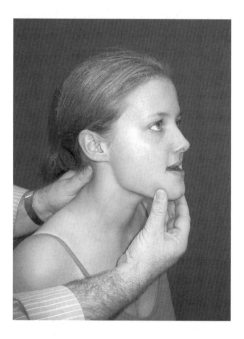

Fig 17.2   Determination of the range of protraction of the mandible.

Depression

With the subject in the same position as above the mandible is pulled inferiorly to open the mouth (Fig. 17.3). The distance between the upper and lower incisors is measured using a plastic rule, one arm of a goniometer or a tape. There should be no lateral deviation of the mandible.

Lateral deviation

With the subject in the same position as above the mandible is pulled laterally (Fig. 17.4). The distance between the upper and lower incisors is measured using a plastic rule, one arm of a goniometer or a tape.

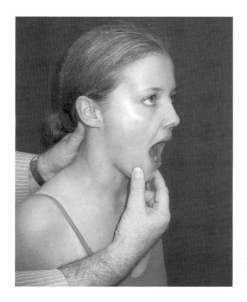

Fig 17.3   Determination of the range of depression of the mandible.

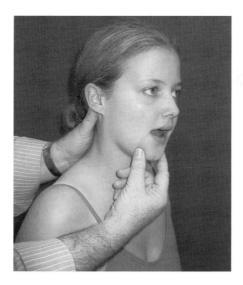

Fig 17.4   Determination of the range of lateral deviation of the mandible.

Section 3

References

Ahlberg A, Moussa M, Al-Nahidi M. (1988) On geographical variations in the normal range of joint motion. *Clinical Orthopaedics* 234; 229–231.

Adler GG, Hoekman RA, Beach DM. (1995) Drop Leg Lachman test – a new test of anterior knee laxity. *American Journal of Sports Medicine* 23; 320–322.

Allander E, Bjornsson OJ, Olafsson O, Sigfusson N, Thorsteinsson J. (1974) Normal range of joint movements in shoulder, hip, wrist and thumb with special reference to side: A comparison between two populations. *International Journal of Epidemiology* 3; 253–261.

American Academy of Orthopaedic Surgeons. (1994) *Joint Motion: Methods of Measuring and Recording* (edited by WB Greene and JD Heckman). American Association of Orthopaedic Surgeons, Illinois.

American Medical Association. (1988) *Guides to the Evaluation of Permanent Impairment, 3rd edition*. American Medical Association.

Aspden RM, Hukins DWL. (1979) The lamina splendens of articular cartilage is an artefact of phase contrast microscopy. *Proceedings of the Royal Society of London (Biology)* 206; 109–113.

Beighton P, Solomon L, Soskolne CL. (1973) Articular mobility in an African population. *Annals of the Rheumatic Diseases* 32; 413–418.

Bell RD, Hoshizaki TB. (1981) Relationships of age and sex with range of motion in seventeen joint actions in humans. *Canadian Journal of Applied Sports Science* 6; 202–206.

Boone DC. *Technique of measurement of joint function.* (1979) (cited in Norkin and White, 1995).

Boone DC, Azen SP, Lin C-N, *et al.* (1978) Reliability of goniometric measurements. *Physical Therapy* 58; 1355–1390.

Boone DC, Azen SP. (1979) Normal range of motion of joints in male subjects. *Journal of Bone and Joint Surgery* 61A; 756–759.

Brumfield RH, Champoux JA. (1984) A biomechanical study of normal functional wrist motion. *Clinical Orthopaedics* 187; 23–25.

Capuano-Pucci D, Rheault W, Ankai J, Bracke M, Day R, Pastrick M. (1991) Intratester and intertester reliability of the cervical range of motion. *Archives of Physical Medicine and Rehabilitation* 72; 338–340.

Cheng JC, Chan PS, Hui PW. (1991) Joint laxity in children. *Journal of Pediatric Orthopaedics* 11; 752–756.

Clarke GR, Willis LA, Fish WW, Nichols PJ. (1975) Preliminary studies in measuring range of motion in normal and painful stiff shoulders. *Rheumatology and Rehabilitation* 14; 39–46.

Downey PA, Fiebert J, Stackpole-Brown JB. (1991) Shoulder range of motion in persons aged sixty and older. *Physical Therapy* 71; S75.

Drews JE, Vraciu JK, Pellino G. (1984) Range of motion of the lower extremities of newborns. *Physical and Occupational Therapy in Pediatrics* 4; 49–62.

Fitzgerald GK, Wynveen KJ, Rheault W, Rothschild B. (1983) Objective assessment with establishment of normal values for lumbar spine range of motion. *Physical Therapy* 63; 1776–1781.

Forero N, Okamura LA, Larson MA. (1989) Normal ranges of hip motion in neonates. *Journal of Pediatric Orthopaedics* 9; 391–395.

Friedman MH, Weisberg J. (1982) Application of orthopaedic principles in evaluation of the temporomandibular joint. *Physical Therapy* 62; 597–603.

Helfet AJ. (1974) Anatomy and biomechanics of movement of the knee joint. In *Disorders of the Knee*, edited by AJ Helfet. JB Lippincott, Philadelphia, pp. 1–17.

Hellebrandt FA, Duvall EN, Moore ML. (1985) The measurement of joint motion. Part III. Reliability of goniometry. *Physical Therapy Review* 65; 1339.

James B, Parker AW. (1989) Active and passive mobility of lower limb joints in elderly men and women. *American Journal of Physical Medicine and Rehabilitation* 68; 162–167.

Jevsevar DS, Riley PO, Hodge WA, Krebs DE. (1993) Knee kinematics and kinetics during locomotion activities of daily living in subjects with knee arthroplasty and in healthy control subjects. *Physical Therapy* 73; 229–239.

Kapandji IA. (1970) *The Physiology of the Joints*. Volume 2, Lower Limb. Churchill Livingstone, Edinburgh.

Kronberg M, Brostrom LA, Soderlund V. (1990) Retroversion of the humeral head in the normal shoulder and its relationship to the normal range of motion. *Clinical Orthopaedics* 253; 113–117.

Laubenthal KN, Smidt GL, Kettelkamp DB. (1972) A quantitative analysis of knee motion during activities of daily living. *Physical Therapy* 52; 34–43.

Livingston LA, Stevenson JM, Olney SJ. (1991) Stairclimbing kinematics on stairs of different dimensions. *Archives of Physical Medicine and Rehabilitation* 72; 398–402.

Ljunggren AE. (1979) Clavicular function. *Acta Orthopaedica Scandinavica* 50; 261–268.

Low JL. (1976) The reliability of joint measurement. *Physiotherapy* 62; 227–229.

Macrae IF, Wright V. (1969) Measurement of back movement. *Annals of the Rheumatic Diseases* 28; 584–589.

Moll JM, Liyanage SP, Wright V. (1972) An objective method to measure lateral spinal flexion. *Rheumatology and Physical Medicine* 11; 225–239.

Moll JM, Wright V. (1971) Normal range of spinal mobility. An objective clinical study. *Annals of the Rheumatic Diseases* 30; 381–386.

Morrey BF, Askew KN, Chao EYS. (1981) A biomechanical study of normal functional elbow motion. *Journal of Bone and Joint Surgery* 63A; 872–877.

Murray MP, Gore DR, Gardner GM, Mollinger LA. (1985) Shoulder motion and muscle strength of normal men and women in two age groups. *Clinical Orthopaedics* 192; 268–273.

Norkin CC, White DJ. (1995) *Measurement of Joint Motion: A Guide to Goniometry*. F.A. Davis Company, Philadelphia.

O'Driscoll SL, Thomenson J. (1982) The cervical spine. *Clinics in Rheumatic Diseases* 8; 617–630.

Phelps E, Smith LJ, Hallum A. (1985) Normal range of hip motion of infants between nine and 24 months of age. *Developmental Medicine and Child Neurology* 27; 785–792.

Poulis S, Poulis I, Soames RW. (2000) Torque characteristics of the ankle plantarflexors and dorsiflexors during eccentric and concentric contraction in healthy young males. *Isokinetics and Exercise Science* 8; 195–202.

Poulis S, Soames RW. Unpublished observations.

Roaas A, Andersson GB. (1982) Normal range of motion of the hip, knee and ankle joint in male subjects, 30–40 years of age. *Acta Orthopaedica Scandinavica* 53; 205–208.

Roach KE, Miles TP. (1991) Normal hip and knee active range of motion: the relationship to age. *Physical Therapy* 71; 656–665.

Safaee-Rad R, Shwedyk E, Quanbury AO, Cooper JE. (1990) Normal functional range of motion of the upper limb joints during performance of three feeding activities. *Archives of Physical Medicine and Rehabilitation* 71; 505–509.

Shereff MJ, Bejjani FJ, Kummer FJ. (1986) Kinematics of the first metatarso-phalangeal joint. *Journal of Bone and Joint Surgery* 68A; 392–398.

Sugahara M, Nakamura M, Sugahara K, Tsuchimoto M, Hirata F, Yukawa K, Ikeda T, Chirifu H. (1981) Epidemiological study on the change of mobility of the thoraco-lumbar spine and body height with age as indices for senility. *Journal of Human Ergology* 10; 49–60.

Svenningsen S, Terjesen T, Auflem M, Berg V. (1989) Hip motion related to age and sex. *Acta Orthopaedica Scandinavica* 60; 97–100.

Tucci SM, Hicks JE, Gross EG, Campbell W, Danoff J. (1986) Cervical motion assessment: a new simple and accurate method. *Archives of Physical Medicine and Rehabilitation* 67; 225–230.

Watanabe H, Ogata K, Amano T, Okabe T. (1979) The range of joint motions of the extremities in healthy Japanese people: the difference according to age. *Journal of the Japanese Orthopaedic Association* 53; 275–281.

Walker JM, Sue D, Miles-Elkousy N, Ford G, Trevelyan H. (1984) Active mobility of the extremities in older subjects. *Physical Therapy* 64; 919–923.

Waugh KG, Minkel JL, Parker R, Coon VA. (1983) Measurement of selected hip, knee, and ankle joint motions in newborns. *Physical Therapy* 63; 1616–1621.

Youdas JW, Carey JR, Garrett TR. (1991) Reliability of measurements of cervical spine range of motion: comparison of three methods. *Physical Therapy* 71; 98–104.

Youdas JW, Carey JR, Garrett TR. (1992) Normal range of motion of the cervical spine. An initial goniometric study. *Physical Therapy* 72; 770–780.

Youm Y, Gillespie TE, Flatt AE, Sprague BL. (1978) Kinematic investigation of normal MCP joint. *Journal of Biomechanics* 11; 109–118.

Youm Y, Yoon YS. (1979) Analytical development in investigation of wrist kinematics. *Journal of Biomechanics* 12; 613–621.

Bibliography

Americal Academy of Orthopaedic Surgeons. (1994) *The Clinical Measurement of Joint Motion* (edited by WB Greene and JD Heckman). American Academy of Orthopaedic Surgeons, Illinois.

Norkin CC, White DJ. (1995) *Measurement of Joint Motion: A Guide to Goniometry.* F.A. Davis Company, Philadelphia.

Palastanga N, Field D, Soames RW. (2002) *Anatomy and Human Movement: Structure and Function, 4th edition.* Butterworth–Heinemann, Oxford.

Index

Note: page numbers in *italics* refer to figures, those in **bold** to tables.